AF522274

A-Z
VETERINARY SCIENCE

A-Z VETERINARY SCIENCE

James Prarera

CENTRUM PRESS
NEW DELHI-110002 (INDIA)

CENTRUM PRESS
H.O.: 4360/4, Ansari Road, Daryaganj,
New Delhi-110 002 (India)
Ph.: 23278000, 23261597
B.O.: No. 1015, Ist Main Road, BSK IIIrd Stage
IIIrd Phase, IIIrd Block,
Bangalore - 560 085 (India)
Tel.: 080-41723429
Visit us at: www.centrumpress.com

A-Z Veterinary Science

First Edition, 2009
ISBN 978-93-80106-40-3

PRINTED IN INDIA

Printed at Salasar Imaging Systems, Delhi-110035 (India)

Contents

Preface

Veterinary research has historically played an important role in the improvement of health and welfare of all animals, including humans. Veterinary scientists are often at the forefront of research in human diseases because many human pathogens have their origins in animal hosts. Moreover, animal models of disease have been used to elucidate the underlying mechanisms of many diseases in humans and other animals.

In addition to its many contributions to human health, veterinary research-by targeting the prevention and control of agricultural, domestic, wild and aquatic animal diseases-contributes to the quality of human life. Food-animal health, for example, secures a safe and economic food supply for the human population. Veterinary research is also essential to the health and increased longevity of service and companion animals and thereby reduces stress in both animals and owners.

Despite the increasing demands on veterinary research, however, its workforce has not increased. The types and priorities of resources dedicated to human and animal health must be reevaluated to address the greatly increased demands on research in the veterinary community.

Author

Chapter 1

Veterinary Science

Veterinary science is the study, diagnosis, treatment and prevention of disease in animals both as individuals and as groups. There is also a key role for members of the profession as guardians of human health in the context of disease transmission from animal or animal products to man.

HISTORICAL AND CURRENT PERSPECTIVE

Once early man had moved from hunting to herding he had an interest in the health and husbandry of his stock. By the time of the ancient civilisations there is evidence of close interaction between man and animals in contexts which are still familiar today including the use of animals for production, draught and war and, increasingly, as human companions. The first book of the modern era devoted to veterinary medicine, 'Artis Veterinariae', was produced by Publius Vegetius Renatus in the second half of the 5th century.

The 'veterinarii' were the animal doctors of ancient Rome, and the word came back into use in the 17th and 18th centuries as the veterinary profession emerged from its origins amongst the farriers. By the 18th century several veterinary texts had been published and the first veterinary school in Europe was established at Lyon in 1762. The first to be established in the United Kingdom was the Royal Veterinary College in 1792.

Although the term 'veterinary surgeon' is widely used within the UK, the term 'veterinarian' is employed here. The veterinary workplace has changed in the last century with less emphasis on the horse (especially as a draught animal), an increasing emphasis on companion animals kept for pleasure, and greater veterinary involvement in production animals, public health and food hygiene. The role of the profession in protecting the health and welfare of more diverse species groups such as laboratory animals, zoological collections, wildlife and, indeed, the contribution to conservation of endangered species, continues to grow.

There is also an increasing body of specialists, both in individual species and in disciplines which cut across species groups, as opportunities for training and the demand for specialist services have grown. The comparative approach of veterinary science will continue to provide insight and support for basic scientists and contribute to the understanding of human disease. The beginning of the 21st century finds the veterinary profession and its work held in high esteem by the general public and a source of considerable interest, with unprecedented exposure of veterinary matters in the popular media. Veterinarians are regarded as guardians of animal health and welfare, and the veterinary schools have a responsibility to continue to produce graduates in whom the public will have confidence.

The sustained public appeal of veterinary work has led to a level of demand for places on veterinary courses which far exceed supply. This demand enables the schools to select strongly motivated, high achievers with entry qualifications among the highest in UK university courses. Most applicants are attracted in the first instance by the prospect of veterinary clinical practice with its unique combination of science, art, practical skills, human-animal and interpersonal interaction. However, an increasing number follow other career paths as they become aware of the diverse opportunities provided by a veterinary degree.

Challenges to Today's Veterinary Medicine

Today, the veterinary profession is confronted with a different set of problems compared with the middle of last century. Now, veterinarians often have to deal with herds or regions remaining diseased after lengthy disease control campaigns. In addition, it is considered necessary to take into account the economic aspects of disease control through the use of benefit/cost analyses of disease control campaigns. Costly multi-factorial *disease complexes* such as mastitis or cattle lameness have become quite common. In addition, old, emerging or new *diseases* with complex aetiologies pose a difficult challenge for the profession. Veterinarians have to respond to the challenges posed by problems such as BSE, FMD and antimicrobial resistance. All these problems require identification, quantification and intensive examination of multiple, directly or indirectly causal, and often interacting, disease determinants.

Veterinary epidemiology and evidence-based veterinary medicine provide overlapping sets of tools which can be used to approach these new challenges. In clinical practice, there is now a daily need for valid, up-to-date information about diagnosis, therapy and prevention. This situation is complicated by the inadequacy of traditional sources for this type of information, since they may be out-of-date, they are frequently wrong, it may be ineffective (didactic CPD), too overwhelming in volume, or too variable in validity. In addition, the clinician

has to deal with the disparity between diagnostic skills and clinical judgement (increasing with experience) on the one hand and up-to-date knowledge and clinical performance (declining with time) on the other. The fact that he/she has insufficient time to examine the animal patient and to practice CPD further complicates the situation.

VETERINARY EPIDEMIOLOGY

Veterinary epidemiology deals with the investigation of diseases, productivity and animal welfare in populations. It is used to describe the frequency of disease occurrence and how disease, productivity and welfare are affected by the interaction of different factors or determinants. This information is then used to manipulate such determinants in order to reduce the frequency of disease occurrence. Veterinary epidemiology is a holistic approach aimed at co-ordinating the use of different scientific disciplines and techniques during an investigation of disease or impaired productivity or welfare. The field of veterinary epidemiology can be divided into different components.

One of its essential foundations is the collection of data, which then has to be analysed using qualitative or quantitative approaches in order to formulate causal hypotheses. As part of the quantitative approach to epidemiological analysis, epidemiological investigations involving field studies or surveys are being conducted and models of epidemiological problems can be developed. The ultimate goal is to control a disease problem, reduce productivity losses and improve animal welfare.

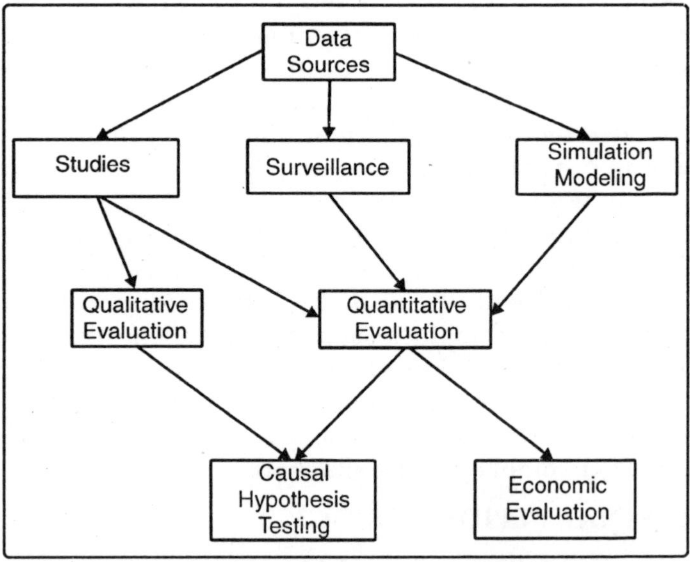

Fig. Components of Veterinary Epidemiology

Measurement of Disease Frequency and Production

One of the most fundamental tasks in epidemiological research is the quantification of the disease occurrence. This can be done simply on the basis of *counts* of individuals which are infected, diseased, or dead. This information will be useful for estimating workload, cost, or size of facilities to provide health care. More commonly, *counts* are expressed as a *fraction* of the number of animals capable of experiencing infection, disease or death. These types of quantities are used by epidemiologists to express the *probability* of becoming infected, diseased or dying for populations with different numbers of individuals (= populations at risk).

From a mathematical perspective, frequency of disease occurrence can be expressed through *static* or *dynamic* measures. *Static measures* include proportions and ratios. A *proportion* is a fraction in which the numerator is included within the denominator. It is dimensionless, ranging from 0 to 1 and is often expressed as a percentage (x 100). The *ratio* is a fraction in which the numerator is not included in the denominator and it can be with or without dimension.

Dynamic measures include *rates* which represent the instantaneous change in one quantity per unit change in another quantity (usually time). They are not dimensionless and do not have a finite upper bound. Measures of disease frequency can be based only on new (=incident) cases of disease or do not differentiate between old and new disease.

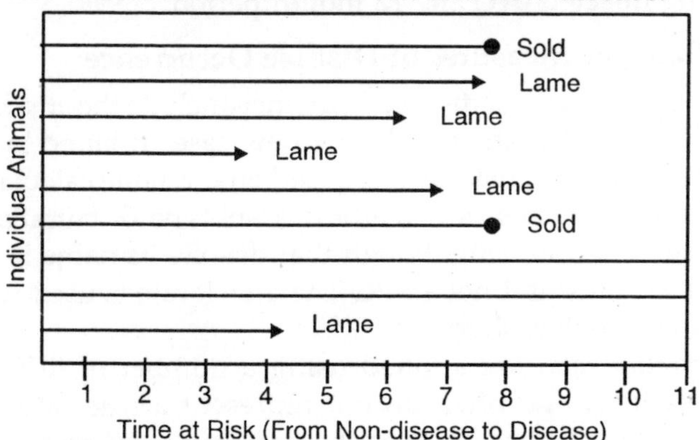

Fig. Incidence of Disease

Figure shows the principles behind incidence measures. They are derived from data for animals which did not have the disease at the beginning of the study period. These animals are followed over time until they develop the disease (eg become lame) or until the observation period finishes (eg sold or end of study period).

Cumulative incidence

The risk of new disease occurrence is quantified using *cumulative incidence,* also called *incidence risk.* It is defined as the proportion of disease-free individuals developing a given disease over a specified time, conditional on that individual's not dying from any other disease during the period.

Note that animals have to be disease free at the beginning of the observation period to be included in the enumerator or denominator of this calculation. It is interpreted as an individual's risk of contracting disease within the risk period. The quantity is dimensionless, ranges from 0 to 1 and always requires a period referent.

As an example, last year a herd of 121 cattle were tested using the tuberculin test and all tested negative. This year, the same 121 cattle were tested again and 25 tested positive. The cumulative incidence over a period of 12 months would then be calculated as 25/121 which amounts to 0.21. Hence, an individual animal within this herd had a 21% chance of becoming infected over the 12 month period.

Miscellaneous Measures of Disease Occurrence

Other measures of disease frequency include the *attack rate* which is defined as the number of new cases divided by the initial population at risk. As it is based on the same calculation as cumulative incidence it really is a subtype of cumulative incidence. It is confusing though that despite its name it is in fact a probability and not a rate. The attack rate is used when the period at risk is short.

Mortality rates are applied using a number of different interpretations, and often do not represent a true rate. The *crude mortality rate* has death as the outcome of interest and is calculated analogous to incidence density. The *cause-specific mortality rate* is estimated for specific causes of death and also calculated analogous to incidence density.

Case fatality rate represents the proportion of animals with a specific disease that die from it. It is a risk measure, not a rate, and is used to describe the impact of epidemics or the severity of acute disease.

Time to the occurrence of an event such as death or onset of clinical disease can be estimated for many epidemiological data sets describing repeated observations on the same sample of animals. This type of data can be summarised using for example mean survival time. This particular method has the disadvantage that the estimate will depend on the length of the time period over which data was collected. If the interval is too short, survival time is likely to be estimated incorrectly, as only individuals who experienced the event of interest can be included in the calculation.

As an alternative, it is possible to calculate an incidence density by using person-years of observation in the denominator and number of events in the enumerator. But this calculation assumes that the rate at which the event occurs is constant throughout the period of study. The most appropriate technique for this data is based on the *survivor* and *hazard function*. The survivor function (=cumulative survival probability) is a functional representation of the proportion of individuals not dying or becoming diseased beyond a given time at risk.

It can be interpreted as the probability of remaining alive for a specific length of time. The survival function is often summarized using the *median survival time* which is the time at which 50% of individuals at risk have failed (died or became diseased). The *hazard function* (=instantaneous failure rate, force of mortality, conditional mortality rate, age specific failure rate) is calculated by dividing the conditional probability of an individual dying or becoming diseased during a specific time interval provided it has not died or become diseased prior to that time divided by the specified *time interval*. This parameter does represent a rate expressing the potential of failing at time t per unit time given survival up until time t.

In the context of survival data, *censoring* is an extremely important concept. In the case of *right censoring*, individuals are lost to follow-up or are not dead/diseased at the end of the follow-up period. This particular type of censoring can be easily accounted for in survival analysis by excluding them from the denominators of the calculations following their departure from the population at risk. With *left censoring*, beginning of the time at risk is not known, and the commonly used analysis techniques cannot take account of this type of censoring. An example calculation for survival data is presented in Figure Animal A survived for 4 months, animal B survived the whole period of 12 months and animal C was removed from the population after 7 months. The number of survivors is based on the actual number of animals still alive after a given time period.

The value for the cohort is used as the denominator for calculation of cumulative survival. The number is adjusted for censored observations. The failures represents the number of deaths during a particular time interval. And the hazard rate is the probability of death per unit time (one month in this case).

STANDARDISATION OF RISK

A crude risk estimate summarises the effects of the specific risk and the subgroup distribution. But in the presence of a confounding factor a crude risk estimate may distort the true pattern. In such a situation, patterns of disease should be described using host-attribute specific risk estimates (e.g. age, sex). For each level of the attribute a separate stratum is formed and stratum-specific risk estimates are calculated. Summary figures can be produced using *standardised* or *adjusted risk* estimates. The two main methods available to perform these calculations are *direct* and *indirect standardisation.*

Direct standardization

Direct standardization involves weighting a set of observed category specific risk estimates according to a *standard* distribution. First, stratum-specific risk rates are calculated. Then a *standard* population distribution is estimated and the proportion of the standard population in each stratum calculated.

The direct adjusted risk rate estimate is obtained as the sum of the products across the strata between the proportion of the *standard* population in stratum *i* and the observed risk rate estimate in stratum *i* in the *study* population. As an example, the mortality in humans in 1963 was compared between Sweden and Panama. In this particular year, Sweden had a population size of 7.496.000 and 73.555 deaths resulting in a *mortality rate* of 0.0098 per year.

Panama had a population size of 1.075.000 with 7871 deaths giving a *mortality rate* of 0.0073 per year. Based on these figures it appeared that life in Sweden was more risky than in Panama. It becomes apparent that in his comparison the confounding factor was the difference in age structure between the two populations.

Sweden had a much lower mortality in young people, but because it had a large proportion of old people this effect did not come through in the aggregated analysis. After adjustment for differences in age structure it turns out that mortality was higher in Panama with 0.0162 per year than it was in Sweden with 0.015 per year.

Indirect standardisation

An alternative approach to standardisation of risk estimates is called *indirect standardisation*. In this case, a *standard* population does not supply the weighting distribution, but a set of stratum-specific risk estimates which are then weighted to the distribution of the *study* population. This technique is used if stratum-specific risk estimates are not available.

But in order to be able to use the method, stratum-specific risk estimates for the *standard* population and the frequency of the adjusting factor in the *study* population have to be available.

As a first step, the expected number of cases is calculated on the basis of the sum of the products between stratum-specific rates for the *standard* population and the total number of individuals in each stratum in the *study* population.

The standardised morbidity or mortality ratio (SMR) is calculated using the number of observed cases divided by the number of expected cases, and the indirect adjusted risk is obtained from multiplying the overall observed risk in the *study* population with the SMR.

ANALYTICAL EPIDEMIOLOGY

The major aims of epidemiology are to *describe* the health status of populations, to *explain* the aetiology of diseases, to *predict* disease occurrence and to *control* the distribution of disease. An understanding of causal relationships is the basis of the last three objectives.

Such associations between causes and disease occurrence can be discovered through individual *case studies*, by experimental *laboratory studies* and by *field studies*. *Case studies* focusing on individual sick animals have long been at the centre of clinical knowledge. They are based on direct personal observations relating to anatomical structure and physiological function, which can be quantified and are systematic but still largely qualitative. While these observations can be extremely intensive and detailed their disadvantage is their subjectivity and the possibly extreme variation between cases. In the *laboratory experiment* - the classic experiment- great precision in measurements and optimal control of influencing variables can be achieved resulting in sound inferences.

The disadvantage is that it is usually not possible to represent the myriad of factors affecting disease occurrence in the natural environment of the animal and it may be difficult to work with sufficient numbers of animals to represent true variation between animals in the natural population. A *field study* is conducted in the natural environment of the animals and measurements are made on sick as well as healthy animals. The differences between sick and healthy animals can be described with respect to the frequency of presence or absence of potential risk factors. With this type of study, animals are exposed to all the known and unknown environmental factors present in their natural environment.

Field research is *empirical* and involves measurement of variables, estimation of population parameters and statistical testing of hypotheses. It is of a *probabilistic nature* in that as a result of a population study it will not be possible to predict with certainty which animal will develop a particular disease given the presence of certain risk factors. But it will be possible to predict how many cases of the disease will occur in the population in the future. Field research involves comparisons among groups in order to estimate the magnitude of an *association* between a putatively causal factor and a disease. The objective is to assess if there is the potential of a cause-effect relationship between a single or multiple risk factors and the disease.

The interrelatedness of phenomena within a biological system complicates the situation for an investigator who will always have to select a segment of the system for the investigation. Attempting to isolate the segment from the rest of the system can result in an outcome which does not represent the real situation in the system anymore.

Analytical epidemiology is aimed at determining the *strength, importance* and *statistical significance* of epidemiological associations. The process typically begins with data collection and eventually leads to data analysis and interpretation. The data collection can be based on a *survey* or a *study*. Both terms are often used interchangeably. A *survey* typically involves *counting* members of an aggregate of units and *measuring* their characteristics. In contrast, a *study* is aimed at comparison of different groups and investigation of cause-effect relationships.

Both designs can be based on a *census* where all members of the population are included thus allowing exact measurement of variables of interest, or alternatively on a *sample* where a subset of the population is included, thereby providing only estimates of the variables of interest.

EPIDEMIOLOGICAL STUDIES

Epidemiological studies are broadly categorised into *non-observational* (or *experimental* studies) and *observational* studies. The first group includes clinical trials or intervention studies and the basic principle is that the design of the study involves deliberately changing population parameters and assessing the effect. With this type of study an attempt is made to simplify observation by *creating* suitable conditions for the study. The second group assumes that the study does not interfere with the population characteristics.

Here, the investigator is only allowed to *select* suitable

conditions for the study. *Observational studies* can be further categorised into *prospective cohort* studies and *retrospective* studies as well as *cross-sectional* studies. *Retrospective studies* include case-control and retrospective cohort studies. Another type of observational study is the *longitudinal* study which is a mix between prospective cohort and repeated cross-sectional studies. Within the group of observational studies mixtures of study designs are common, such as for example the case-cohort study. The *case series* is a separate group of studies and frequently used in a clinical context.

This type of study typically involves dividing a group of animals into a subgroup which is being *treated* and another subgroup which is being left *untreated* and acts as a control. The decision to treat an animal or leave it untreated is typically based on random allocation - *randomisation*. After a period of time the status with respect to a response variable (e.g. disease status) is assessed for each animal.

Summary measures of the response are then compared between both subgroups. Differences in the summary values suggest the presence of an effect of the *treatment* on the response variable. Non-observational or experimental studies can be conducted as *laboratory experiments* or as *field studies* such as *clinical trials*. The latter are usually used to evaluate therapeutic or preventive effects of particular interventions, but are also useful to investigate etiologic relationships.

The *non-observational study* provides the researcher with effective control over the study situation. If the sample size is large enough a well-designed experiment will limit the effect of unwanted factors even if they are not measurable. Control of factors other than the treatment which are likely to have an effect on disease can be achieved by using them to define homogeneous subgroups with respect to the status of these variables - *blocking* or *matching*- within which treatment is then allocated randomly.

The possibility to have excessive control over the study situation can become a weakness of the non-observational approach as it may not be representative of the real situation in the biological system anymore. *Clinical trials* are considered the method of choice for investigation of causal hypotheses about the effectiveness of preventive measures, and compared with the other types of field studies they can provide the strongest evidence about causality.

There is less opportunity for systematic error compared with the observational studies. Amongst their disadvantages are the following characteristics. They require large groups, are costly, bias may be introduced through selection error and the required duration can be long if disease incidence is low.

SAMPLING OF ANIMAL POPULATIONS

The main objectives of sampling are to provide data which will allows making inferences in relation about a larger population on the basis of examining a sample in relation to for example presence/absence of animal disease or other parameters of interest. Inferences might relate to proving that disease is not present, to detecting presence of disease or establishing the level of disease occurrence. The objective could also be to describe levels of milk production in a population of dairy cattle or more generally provide a descriptive analysis of an animal production system for example in an African country.

DATA SOURCES

Any *data sources* for epidemiological analyses have to be evaluated with respect to their *completeness, validity* and *representativeness*. The data can be collected as part of *routine data collection* which includes laboratory submissions, disease surveillance programmes, industry- or farm/ bureau based data recording systems and abattoirs.

More recently, *structured data collection* has been found to provide a more effective way for regular monitoring of disease / production. And finally, data can be collected as part of *epidemiological studies*. Data which is based on *laboratory submissions* is useful for detecting disease.

It can become the basis of case series and case control studies. It does not provide sufficient data to allow prevalence estimation, because the enumerator and denominator are likely to both be biased. In isolation, laboratory submissions do not provide information about causation !!!! They are also not useful for evaluation of therapies or economic effects.

The data collection process can include the whole population of interest (=*census*) or it can be restricted to a *sample*. The latter has the advantage over the *census* that results can be obtained more quickly. A sample is less expensive to collect, and sample results may be more accurate as it is possible to make more efficient use of resources. In addition, *probability samples* result in probability estimates which allow inferences to be used for other populations.

Heterogeneity in the results can be reduced by targeted sampling of particular sub-groups within the population. Involvement of the whole population such as is necessary for a census may not be possible due to logistic or administrative problems, so that sampling becomes the method of choice. The sampling process can be described using the following terminology. The *target population* represents the population at risk. The population effectively sampled is called the *study population*. Frequently, the target population is not completely accessible, so that it differs to a possibly unknown extent from the study population.

It is then necessary to use common sense judgement in order to assess the representativeness of the study population in relation to the target population. The *sampling frame* lists all sampling units in the study population, and is an essential requirement for probability sampling. *Sampling units* are the individual members of the sampling frame.

INTERPRETATION OF DIAGNOSTIC TESTS

UNCERTAINTY AND THE DIAGNOSTIC PROCESS

The duties of the veterinary profession include "to maintain and enhance the health, productivity and well-being of all animals" and "to prevent and relieve animal suffering". In order to fulfill this duty, the veterinarian has to be able to diagnose disease or production problems as well as identify possible causes.

Diagnosis is the basis for a decision, such as whether to treat (or implement a programme) or to do nothing, to further evaluate, euthanase or to wait. The tools which the veterinarian uses to come to a diagnosis include factual knowledge, experience, intuition as well as diagnostic tests. Correct use of these four mechanisms maximises the probability of a correct diagnosis. The uncertainty with regard to the effect of a treatment on a patient's health made the ancient Greeks call medicine a *stochastic art.*

Clearly, the main task of any veterinarian is to deal with the uncertainty of both, diagnosis and the outcome of treatment. It has been shown in studies of the medical profession that fear of personal inadequacy and failure in reacting to this uncertainty is a common characteristic among physicians. This has become an even more important problem as our society becomes increasingly specialized and technological, relying on science rather than religion or magic to explain uncertainties.

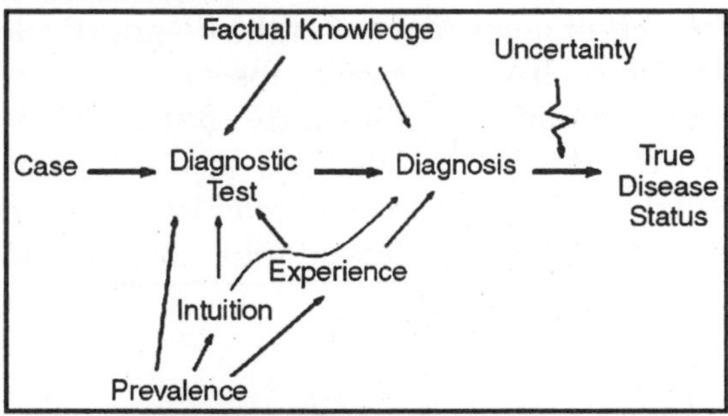

Fig. Factors Influencing Veterinary

In this context, one should be aware of two major paradigms used to explain biological processes. The *mechanistic paradigm* assumes deterministic causation, and experiments are conducted to develop rules or laws according to which nature is thought to 'work'. Obviously, the client in a diagnostic situation does prefer this kind of interpretation, as it increases confidence in the diagnostic and the therapeutic process.

The *probabilistic paradigm* on the other hand assumes probabilistic causation. Diagnostic and therapeutic procedures are seen as gambles and it is recognised that the decision making process incorporates subjective judgement. The conclusion has to be though that given our incomplete understanding of biological systems and the presence of true biological variation, in veterinary diagnosis one must be content to end not in certainties, but rather statistical probabilities.

The outcome of the *diagnostic process* is a statement as to whether an animal is considered normal or not normal. This could relate to disease or infection status as well as to productive performance or quality of life from an animal welfare perspective.

DIAGNOSTIC TESTS

The diagnostic test is a more or less objective method for reducing *diagnostic uncertainty*. As the consequential decisions are typically dichotomous (treat or do not), the outcome of the diagnostic process often is interpreted as a dichotomous variable as well, such as the animal having or not having the disease. The unit of measurement of the diagnostic device can be dichotomous, such as presence or absence of bacteria, which facilitates interpretation significantly. But if the diagnostic device measures on a continuous scale, such as serum antibody levels or somatic cell counts, a *cut-off value* has to be determined so that the result can be condensed into a dichotomous scale.

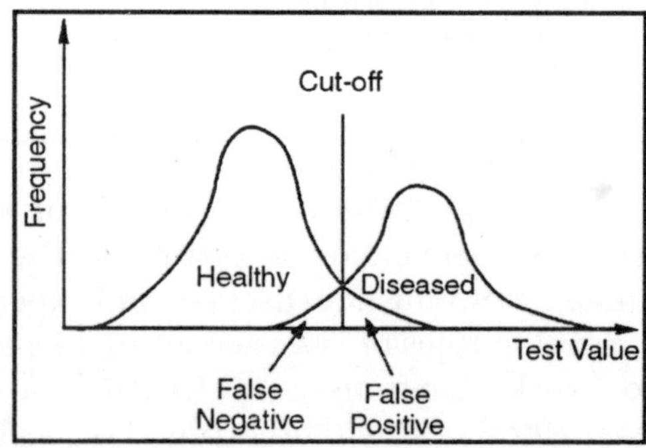

Fig. Test Result Measured on Continuous Scale

Given a clinical measurement on a continuous scale, the problem with any cut-off point is that it is likely to result in overlap between healthy and diseased individuals with regard to test results. The consequences of this situation are that uncertainty in addition to any other potential sources of measurement error (such as operator error) is being introduced. It is desirable to quantify this relationship between diagnostic test result and "true" disease status so that the clinician can take account of this uncertainty when interpreting test results.

The performance of a diagnostic method can be described using the *accuracy* which refers to the closeness between test result and "true" clinical state, the *bias* which is a measure of the systematic deviation from "true" clinical state, and the *precision* or *repeatability* representing the degree of fluctuation of a test series around a central measurement.

Any evaluation of diagnostic tests needs a measure of the "true" condition of individuals to compare with which is usually called the *gold standard*. Most of the time it is impossible to define with 100% accuracy what the true diagnosis should be. There may also be disagreement amongst experts such as for example in the case of mastitis where the presence of the particular pathogen *or* the presence of an inflammatory response in the udder could be defined as the gold standard.

Chapter 2

Animals Nutrition

FEEDING BEHAVIOUR

Buffaloes are strict grazers and only browse when feed is utterly scarce. Normally, buffaloes graze during the day. In case of extremely high ambient temperatures, grazing takes place in the morning and afternoon and sometimes during night time. Buffaloes graze more and better than cattle. Thereby they consume more feed and nutrients per kg of body weight than cattle do.

Newborn calves suckle their mothers within two hours of birth. Normal suckling frequency is approximately 6 to 8 times per day. The calves start to nibble grass at 3 to 4 weeks of age, although they are not actually grazing until after a few weeks more. When the calves have reached two months of age, forage starts to become more important than previously and soon most of the nutrient intake comes from forage rather than milk. Natural weaning of calves is usually within a year or before its mother's next parturition.

NUTRITION FOR HORSE

Equine nutrition refers to the feeding of horses, ponies, mules, donkeys, and other equines. Correct and balanced nutrition is a critical component of proper horse care. Horses are herbivores, a type of non-ruminant known as a "hind-gut fermentor." What this means is that horses have only one stomach, similar to humans. However, unlike humans, they also have to digest plant fibre that comes from grass and hay. Therefore, unlike ruminants, who digest fibre in plant matter by use of a multichambered stomach, horses use bacterial fermentation that occurs in the organ known as the *cecum* (or *caecum*) to break down cellulose.

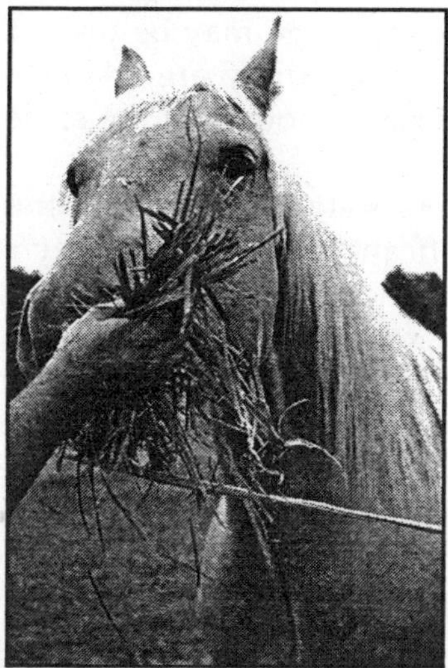

Fig. Grass is a Natural Source of Nutrition for a Horse

In practical terms, horses prefer to eat small amounts of food steadily throughout the day, as they do in nature when grazing on pasture. Although this is not always possible with modern stabling practices and human schedules that favour feeding horses twice a day, it is important to remember the underlying biology of the animal when determining what to feed, how often, and in what quantities. The digestive system of the horse is somewhat delicate.

Because horses are unable to regurgitate food, except from the esophagus, if they overeat or eat something poisonous, vomiting is not an option. They also have a long, complex large intestine and a balance of beneficial bacteria in their cecum that can be upset by rapid changes in feed. Because of these factors, they are very susceptible to colic, which is a leading cause of death in horses. Therefore, horses require clean, high-quality feed, provided at regular intervals, and may become ill if subjected to abrupt changes in their diets.

Horses are also sensitive to molds and toxins. For this reason, they must never be fed contaminated fermentable materials such as lawn clippings. Fermented silage, sometimes called "haylage" is fed to horses in some places; however, contamination or failure of the fermentation process that allows any mold or spoilage may be toxic. Horses and other members of the *Equidae* family are adapted by evolutionary biology to eating small amounts of the same kind of food all day long.

In the wild, horses ate prairie grasses in semi-arid regions and traveled significant distances each day in order to obtain adequate nutrition. Therefore, their digestive system was made to work best with a small but steady flow of food that does not change much from day to day. Digestion begins in the mouth. First, the animal selects pieces of forage and picks up finer foods, such as grain, with sensitive, prehensile, lips.

The front teeth of the horse, called incisors, clip forage, and food is ground up for swallowing by the premolars and molars. The esophagus carries food to the stomach. The esophagus enters the stomach at an acute angle, creating a one-way valve, with a powerful spincter mechanism at the gastroesophageal junction, which is why horses cannot vomit. The esophagus is also the area of the digestive tract where horses may suffer from choke.

Horses have a relatively small stomach for their size, which limits the amount of feed that can be taken in at one time. The average sized horse has a stomach with a capacity of only four gallons, and works best when it contains about two gallons. One reason continuous foraging or several small feedings per day are better than one or two large meals is because the stomach begins to empty when it is 2/3 full, whether the food in the stomach is processed or not.

The small intestine is 50 to 70 feet long and holds 10 to 12 gallons. This is the major digestive organ where most nutrients are absorbed. Bile from the liver acts here, combined with enzymes from the pancreas and small intestine itself. Equids do not have a gall bladder, so bile flows constantly, another reason for a slow but steady supply of food.

Most nutrition is absorbed into the bloodstream from the small intestine. The cecum is the first section of the large intestine. It is also known as the "water gut" or "hind gut." It is a cul-de-sac pouch, about 4 feet long that holds 7 to 8 gallons. It digests cellulose plant fibre through bacterial fermentation. The reason horses must have their diets changed slowly is so the bacteria in the cecum are able to modify and adapt to the different chemical structure of new feedstuffs. Too abrupt a change in diet can cause colic, as the new food is not properly digested.

The large colon, small colon, and rectum make up the remainder of the large intestine. The large colon is 10-12 feet long and holds up to 20 gallons of semi-liquid matter. Its main purpose it to absorb carbohydrates which were broken down from cellulose in the cecum. Due to its many twists and turns, it is a common place for a type of horse colic called an impaction. The small colon is 10-12 feet long, holds about 5 gallons, is the area where the majority of water is absorbed, and where fecal balls are formed. The rectum is about one foot long, and acts as a holding chamber for waste, which is then expelled from the body via the anus.

Nutrients

Like all animals, equines require five main classes of nutrients to survive: water, energy (primarily in the form of fats and carbohydrates), proteins, vitamins, and minerals.

Water makes up between 62-68 per cent of a horse's body weight and is essential for life. Horses can only live a few days without water, becoming dangerously dehydrated if they lose 8-10 per cent of their natural body water. Therefore, it is critically important to provide access to a fresh, clean, and adequate supply of water. An average 450kg horse drinks 10 to 12 gallons of water per day, more in hot weather, when eating dry forage such as hay, or when consuming high levels of salt, potassium, and magnesium.

Horses drink less water in cool weather or when on lush pasture, which has a relatively higher water content. When under hard work, or if a mare is lactating, water requirements may be as much as four times greater than normal. Though they need a great deal of water, horses spend very little time drinking; usually 1-8 minutes a day, spread out in 2-8 episodes. Water plays an important part in digestion. The forages and grains horses eat are mixed with saliva in the mouth to make a moist bolus that can be easily swallowed. Therefore, horses produce up to 10 gallons of saliva per day.

Nutritional sources of energy are fat and carbohydrates. Protein is a critical building block for muscles and other tissues. Horses that are heavily exercised, growing, pregnant or lactating need increased energy and protein in their diet. However, if a horse has too much energy in its diet and not enough exercise, it can become too high-spirited and difficult to handle.Fat exists in low levels in plants and can be added to increase the energy density of the diet.

Fat has 9 Mcal/kg of energy, which is 2.25 times that of any carbohydrate source. Because equids have no gall bladder to store large quantities of bile, which flows continuously from the liver directly into the small intestine, fat, though a necessary nutrient, is difficult for them to digest and utilize in large quantities. However, they are able digest a greater amount of fat than can cattle. Horses benefit from up to 8 per cent fat in their diets, but more does not always provide a visible benefit. Horses can only have 15 per cent-20 per cent fat in their diet without the risk of developing diarrhea.

Carbohydrates, the main energy source in most rations, are usually fed in the form of hay, grass and grain. Soluble carbohydrates such as starches and sugars are readily broken down to glucose in the small intestine and absorbed. Insoluble carbohydrates, such as fibre (cellulose), are not digested by enzymes, but are fermented by microbes in the cecum and large colon to break down and release their energy sources, the volatile fatty acids.

Soluble carbohydrates are found in nearly every feed source; corn has the highest amount, then barley and oats. Forages normally have only 6 to 8 per cent soluble carbohydrate, but under certain conditions can have up to 30 per cent. Sudden ingestion of large amounts of starch or high sugar feeds can cause colic or laminitis.Protein is used in all parts of the body, especially muscle, blood, hormones, hooves, and hair cells. The main building blocks of protein are amino acids. Alfalfa and other legumes in hay are good sources of protein that can be easily added to the diet. Most adult horses only require 8 to 10 per cent protein in their diet; however, higher protein is important for lactating mares and young growing foals.

Horses that are not subjected to hard work or extreme conditions usually have more than adequate amounts of vitamins in their diet if they are receiving fresh, green, leafy forages. Sometimes a vitamin supplement is needed when feeding low-quality hay, if a horse is under stress (illness, traveling, showing, racing, and so on), or not eating well. Grain has a different balance of nutrients than forage, and so requires specialized supplementation to prevent an imbalance of vitamins and minerals.

Minerals are required for maintenance and function of the skeleton, nerves and muscles. These include calcium, phosphorus, sodium, potassium, and chloride, and are commonly found in most good-quality feeds. Horses also need trace minerals such as magnesium, selenium, copper, zinc and iodine. Normally, if adult animals at maintenance levels are consuming fresh hay or are on pasture, they will receive adequate amounts of minerals in their diet, with the exception of sodium chloride (salt), which needs to be provided, preferably free choice. Some pastures are deficient in certain minerals, especially selenium or copper, and in such situations, deficiency diseases may occur if the horses' feed is not supplemented.

Calcium and phosphorus are needed in a specific ratio of between 1:1 and 2:1. Adult horses can tolerate up to a 5:1 ratio, foals no more than 3:1. A total ration with a higher ratio of phosphorus than calcium is to be avoided. Over time, the imbalance will ultimately lead to bone problems such as osteoporosis.

Foals and young growing horses through their first three to four years have special nutritional needs and require feeds that are balanced with a proper calcium:phosphorus ratio and other trace minerals. A number of skeletal problems may occur in young animals with an unbalanced diet. Hard work increases the need for minerals; sweating depletes sodium, potassium, and chloride from the horse's system. Therefore, supplementation with electrolytes may be required for horses in intense training, especially in hot weather.

Types of Feed

Equids can consume approximately 2 per cent to 2.5 per cent of their body weight in dry feed each day. Therefore, a 1000 lb adult horse could eat up to 25 pounds of food. Foals less than six months of age eat 2 to 4 per cent of their weight each day.Solid feeds are placed into three categories: forages, concentrates (including grain or pelleted rations), and supplements.

Equine nutritionists recommend that 50 per cent or more of the animal's diet by weight should be forages. If a horse is working hard and requires more energy, the use of grain is increased and the percentage of forage decreased so that the horse obtains the energy content it needs for the work it is performing. However, forage amount should never go below 1 per cent of the horse's body weight per day.

Forages, also known as "roughage," are plant materials classified as legumes or grasses, found in pastures or in hay. Often, pastures and hayfields will contain a bland of both grasses and legumes. Nutrients available in forage vary greatly with maturity of the grasses, fertilization, management, and environmental conditions. Grasses are tolerant of a wide range of conditions and contain most necessary nutrients. Some commonly used grasses include timothy, brome, fescue, coastal bermuda, orchard grass, and Kentucky bluegrass.

Legumes such as clover or alfalfa are usually higher in protein, calcium, and energy than grasses. However, they require warm weather and good soil to produce the best nutrients. Legume hays are generally higher in protein than the grass hays. They are also higher in minerals, particularly calcium, but have an incorrect ratio of calcium to phosphorus. Because they are high in protein, they are very desirable for growing horses or those subjected to very hard work, but the calcium:phosphorus ratio must be balanced by other feeds to prevent bone abnormalities.

Hay is a dried mixture of grasses and legumes. It cut in the field and then dried and baled for storage. Hay is most nutritious when it is cut early on, before the seed heads are fully mature and before the stems of the plants become tough and thick. Hay that is very green can be a good indicator of the amount of nutrients in the hay; however, colour should not be used as sole indicator - smell and texture are also important. Hay can be analyzed by many laboratories and that is the most reliable way to tell the nutritional values it contains. Moldy or dusty hay should not be fed to horses, as it is the most common cause of Recurrent airway obstruction, also known as COPD or "heaves."

Hay, particularly alfalfa, is sometimes compressed into pellets or cubes. Processed hay can be of more consistent quality and is more convenient to ship and to store. It is also easily obtained in areas that may be suffering localized hay shortages. However, these more concentrated forms can be overfed and horses are somewhat more prone to choke on them. On the other hand, hay pellets and cubes can be soaked until they break apart into a pulp or thick slurry, and in this state are a very useful source of food for horses with tooth problems such as dental disease, tooth loss due to age, or structural anomalies.

Haylage, also known as *Round bale silage* is a term for grass sealed in airtight plastic bags, a form of forage that is frequently fed in the United Kingdom and continental Europe, but is not often seen in the United States. Because haylage is a type of silage, hay stored in this fashion must remain completely sealed in plastic, as any holes or tears can stop the preservation properties of fermentation and lead to mold or spoilage. Rodents chewing through the plastic can also spoil the hay introducing contamination to the bale.If a rodent dies inside the plastic, the subsequent botulism toxins released can contaminate the entire bale.

Another type of forage sometimes provided to horses is beet pulp, a byproduct left over from the processing of sugar beets, which is high in energy as well as fibre.Sometimes, straw or chaff from cereal grains is fed to animals. However, this is roughage with little nutritional value. It is not recommended by nutritionists as a horse feed, though it is sometimes used as a filler; it can slow down horses who eat their grain too fast, or it can provide additional fibre when the horse must meet most nutritional needs via concentrated feeds. Straw is more often used as a bedding in stalls to absorb wastes.

Whole or crushed grains are the most common form of concentrated feed, sometimes referred to generically as "oats" or "corn" even if those grains are not present, also sometimes called "straights" in the UK.

Oats are the most popular grain for horses. Oats have a lower digestible energy value and higher fibre content than most other grains. They form a loose mass in the stomach that is well suited to the equine digestive system. They are also more palatable and digestible other grains.

Corn, referred to as Maize in the UK, is the second most palatable grain. It provides twice as much digestible energy as an equal volume of oats and is low in fibre. Because of these characteristics, is easy to over-feed corn, causing obesity, so horses are seldom fed corn all by itself. Nutritionists caution horse owners that moldy corn should never be fed because it is poisonous to horses.

Barley is also fed to horses, but needs to be processed to crack the seed hull and allow easier digestibility. It is frequently fed in combination with oats and corn, a mix informally referred to by the acronym "COB" (for Corn, Oats and Barley).

Wheat is generally not used as a concentrate. However, wheat bran is sometimes added to the diet of a horse for supplemental nutrition, usually moistened and in the form of a bran mash. Wheat bran is high in phosphorus, so must be fed carefully so that it does not cause an imbalance in the Ca:P ratio of a ration. Once touted for a laxative effect, this use of bran is now considered unnecessary, as horses, unlike humans, obtain sufficient fibre in their diets from other sources.

Many feed manufacturers combine various grains and add

additional vitamin and mineral supplements to create a complete premixed feed that is easy for owners to feed and of predictable nutritional quality. Some of these prepared feeds are manufactured in pelleted form, others retain the grains in their original form. In many cases molasses as a binder to keep down dust and for increased palatability. Grain mixes with added molasses are usually called "Sweet feed" in the USA and "Coarse mix" in the United Kingdom. Pelleted or *extruded* feeds (sometimes referred to as "nuts" in the UK) may be easier to chew and result in less wasted feed. Horses generally eat pellets as easily as grain. However, pellets are also more expensive, and even "complete" rations do not eliminate the necessity for forage.

The average modern horse on good hay or pasture with light work usually does not need supplements; however, horses subjected to stress due to age, intensive athletic work, or reproduction may need additional nutrition. Extra fat and protein are sometimes added to the horse's diet, along with vitamin and mineral supplements.

Soybean meal is a common protein supplement, and averages about 44 per cent crude protein. The protein in soybean meal is high-quality, with the proper ratio of dietary essential amino acids for equids. Cottonseed meal, Linseed meal, and peanut meal are also used, but are not as common.

Vegetable oil is a common fat source added to a ration. Corn oil is particularly popular, but other oils are used as well. Rice bran is a very good fat supplement that contains 20 per cent fat as well as fibre and other nutrients. Flax seed is another good source of fat, though it must ground up for horses to digest it. Some commercial feed manufacturers now make products containing both flaxseed and rice bran.

There are hundreds, if not thousands of commercially prepared vitamin and mineral supplements on the market, many tailored to horses with specialized needs.

Most horses only need quality forage, water and a salt or mineral block. Grain or other concentrates are often not necessary. But, when grain or other concentrates are fed, quantities must be carefully monitored. To do so, horse feed is measured by weight, not volume. For example, 1 lb. of oats has a different volume than 1 lb. of corn. When continuous access to feed is not possible, it is more consistent with natural feeding behaviour to provide three small feedings per day instead of one or two large ones.

However, even two daily feedings is preferable to only one. To gauge the amount to feed, a weight tape, available at most feed stores, can be used to provide a reasonably accurate estimate of a horse's weight. The tape measures the circumference of the horse's barrel, just behind the withers and elbows, and the tape is calibrated to convert inches or centimeters into approximate pounds or kilograms.

Actual amounts fed vary by the size of the horse, the age of the horse, the climate, and the work to which the animal is put. In addition, genetic factors play a role. Some animals are naturally easy keepers, which means that they can thrive on relatively small amounts of food and are prone to obesity and other health problems if overfed. Others are hard keepers, meaning that they are prone to be thin and require considerably more food to maintain a healthy weight.

Veterinarians are usually a good source for recommendations on appropriate types and amounts of feed for a specific horse. There are also numerous books written on the topic. Feed manufacturers usually offer very specific guidelines for how to select and properly feed products from their company, and in the United States, the local office of the Cooperative Extension Service can provide educational materials and expert recommendations.

Equids always require forage. When possible, nutritionists recommend it be available at all times, at least when doing so does not overfeed the animal and lead to obesity. It is safe to feed a ration that is 100 per cent forage (along with water and supplemental salt), and any feed ration should be at least 50 per cent forage. Hay with alfalfa or other legumes has more concentrated nutrition and so is fed in smaller amounts than grass hay, though many hays have a mixture of both types of plant.

When beet pulp is fed, a ration of 2 to 5 pounds is usually

soaked in water for 3 to 4 hours prior to feeding in order to make it more palatable, and to minimize the risk of choke and other problems. It is usually soaked in a proportion of one part beet pulp to two parts water. Beet pulp is usually fed in addition to hay, but occasionally is a replacement for hay when fed to very old horses who can no longer chew properly.

Some pelleted rations are designed to be a "complete" feed that contains both hay and grain, meeting all the horse's nutritional needs. However, even these rations should have some hay or pasture provided, a minimum of a half-pound of forage for every 100 pounds of horse, in order to keep the digestive system functioning properly and to meet the horse's urge to graze.

Recent studies address the level of various non-structural carbohydrates (NSC), such as fructan, in forages. Too high an NSC level causes difficulties for animals prone to laminitis or equine polysaccharide storage myopathy (EPSM). NSC cannot be determined by looking at forage, but hay and pasture grasses can be tested for NSC levels.

Concentrates, when fed, are recommended to be provided in quantities no greater than 1 per cent of a horse's body weight per day, and preferably in two or more feedings. If a ration needs to contain a higher percent of concentrates, such as that of a race horse, bulky grains such as oats should be used as much as possible; a loose mass of feed helps prevent impaction colic. Peptic ulcers are linked to a too-high concentration of grain in the diet, particularly noticed modern racehorses, where some studies show such ulcers affecting up to 90 per cent of all race horses.

In general, the portion of the ration that should be grain or other concentrated feed is 0 to 10 per cent grain for mature idle horses; between 20 to 70 per cent for horses at work, depending on age, intensity of activity and energy requirements. Concentrates should not be fed to horses within one hour before or after a heavy workout. Concentrates also need to be adjusted to level of performance. Not only can excess grain and inadequate exercise lead to behaviour problems, it may also trigger Equine Exertional

Rhabdomyolysis, or "tying up," in horses prone to the condition.

Horses normally require free access to all the fresh, clean water they want, and to avoid dehydration, should not be kept from water longer than four hours at any one time. However, water may need to be temporarily limited in quantity when a horse is very hot after a heavy workout. As long as a hot horse continues to work, it can drink its fill at periodic intervals, provided that common sense is used and that an overheated horse is not forced to drink from extremely cold water sources.

But when the workout is over, a horse needs to be cooled out and walked for 30—90 minutes before it can be allowed all the water it wants at one time. However, dehydration is also a concern, so some water needs to be offered during the cooling off process. A hot horse will properly rehydrate while cooling off if offered a few swallows of water every three to five minutes while being walked. Sometimes the thirst mechanism does not immediately kick in following a heavy workout, which is another reason to offer periodic refills of water throughout the cooling down period.

Even a slightly dehydrated horse is at higher risk of developing impaction colic. Additionally, dehydration can lead to weight loss because the horse cannot produce adequate amounts of saliva, thus decreasing the amount of feed and dry forage consumed. Thus, it is especially important for horse owners to encourage their horses to drink when there is a risk of dehydration; when horses are losing a great deal of water in hot weather due to strenuous work, or in cold weather due to horses' natural tendency to drink less when in a cold environment. To encourage drinking, owners may add electrolytes to the feed, additives to make the water especially palatable (such as apple juice), or, when it is cold, to warm the water so that it is not at a near-freezing temperature.

Special Feeding Issues for Ponies

Ponies and miniature horses are usually easy keepers and need less feed than full-sized horses. This is not only because they are smaller, but also, because they evolved under harsher living conditions than horses, they use feed more efficiently. Ponies easily become obese from overfeeding and therefore are at high risk for colic, Equine Metabolic Syndrome, and, especially, laminitis. Fresh grass is a particular danger to ponies; they can develop laminitis in as little as one hour of grazing on lush pasture.

It is important to track the weight of a pony carefully, by use of a weight tape. Forages may be fed based on weight, at a rate of about 1 pound of forage for every 100 pounds. Forage, along with water and a salt and mineral block, is all most ponies require.

If a hard-working pony needs concentrates, a ratio of no more than 30 per cent concentrates to 70 per cent forage is recommended. Concentrates designed for horses, with added vitamins and minerals, will often provide insufficient nutrients at the small serving sizes needed for ponies. Therefore, if a pony requires concentrates, feed and supplements designed specially for ponies should be used. In the UK, extruded pellets designed for ponies are sometimes called "pony nuts.".

Special Feeding Issues for Mules and Donkeys

Like ponies, mules and donkeys are also very hardy and generally need less concentrated feed than horses. Mules need less protein than horses and do best on grass hay with a vitamin and mineral supplement. If mules are fed concentrates, they only need about half of what a horse requires. Like horses, mules require fresh, clean water, but are less likely to over-drink when hot.

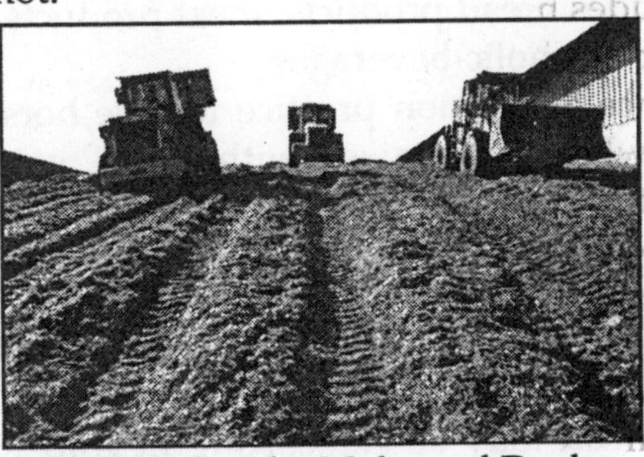

Fig. Grass hay for Mules and Donkey

Donkeys, like mules, need less protein and more fibre than horses. They do best when allowed to consume small amounts of food over long periods, as is natural for them in an arid climate. They can meet their nutritional needs on 6 to 7 hours of grazing per day on average dryland pasture that is not stressed by drought. If they are worked long hours or do not have access to pasture, they require hay or a similar dried forage, with no more than a 1:4 ratio of legumes to grass. They also require salt and mineral supplements, and access to clean, fresh water. Like ponies and mules, in a lush climate, donkeys are prone to obesity and are at risk of laminitis.

Many people like to feed horses special treats such as carrots, sugar cubes, peppermint candies or specially manufactured horse "cookies." Horses do not need treats, and due to the risk of colic or choke, many horse owners do not allow their horses to be given treats. There are also behavioural issues that some horses may develop if given too many treats, particularly a tendency to bite if hand-fed, and for this reason many horse trainers and riding instructors discourage the practice.

However, if treats are allowed, carrots and compressed hay pellets are common, nutritious, and generally not harmful. Apples are also acceptable, though it is best if they are first cut into slices. Horse "cookies" are often specially manufactured out of ordinary grains and some added molasses. They generally will not cause nutritional problems when fed in small quantities. However, many types of human foods are potentially dangerous to a horse and should not be fed. This includes bread products, meat products, candy, and carbonated or alcoholic beverages.

It was once a common practice to give horses a weekly *bran mash* of wheat bran mixed with warm water and other ingredients. It is still done regularly in some places. While a warm, soft meal is a treat many horses enjoy, and was once considered helpful for its laxative effect, it is not nutritionally necessary. An old horse with poor teeth may benefit from food softened in water, a mash may help provide extra hydration, and a warm meal may be comforting in cold weather, but horses have far more fibre in their regular diet than do humans, and so any assistance from bran is unnecessary. There is also a risk that too much wheat bran may provide excessive phosphorus, unbalancing the diet, and a feed of unusual contents fed only once a week could trigger a bout of colic.

All hay and concentrated feeds must kept dry and free of mold, rodent feces and other types of contamination that may cause illness in horses. Feed kept outside or otherwise exposed to moisture can develop mold quite quickly. Due to fire hazards, hay is often stored under an open shed or under a tarp, rather than inside a horse barn itself, but should be kept under some kind of cover.

Concentrates take up less storage space, are less of a fire hazard, and are usually kept in a barn or enclosed shed. A secure door or latched gate between the animals and any feed storage area is critical. Horses accidentally getting into stored feed and eating too much at one time is a common but preventable way that horses develop colic or laminitis.

It is also important to never give a horse feed that was contaminated by the remains of a dead animal, it is a potential source of botulism. This is not an uncommon situation. For example, mice and birds can get into poorly stored grain and be trapped; hay bales sometimes accidentally contain snakes, mice, or other small animals that were caught in the baling machinery during the harvesting process.

Horses can become anxious or stressed if there are long periods of time between meals. They also do best when they are fed on a regular schedule, they are creatures of habit and easily upset by changes in routine. When horses are in a herd, their behaviour is hierarchical; the higher-ranked animals in the herd eat and drink first. Low-status animals, who eat last, may not get enough food, and if there is little available feed, higher-ranking horses may keep lower-ranking ones from eating at all.

Therefore, unless a herd is on pasture that meets the nutritional needs of all individuals, it is important to either feed horses separately, or spread feed out in separate areas to be sure all animals get roughly equal amounts of food to eat.

In some situations where horses are kept together, they may still be placed into separate herds, depending on nutritional needs; overweight horses are kept separate from thin horses so that rations may be adjusted accordingly.

Horses' teeth continually erupt throughout their life, are worn down as they eat, and can develop uneven wear patterns that can interfere with chewing. For this reason, horses need a dental examination at least once a year, and particular care must be paid to the dental needs of older horses. The process of grinding off uneven wear patterns on a horse's teeth is called *floating* and can be performed by a veterinarian or a specialist in equine dentistry.Diet and Nutrition for Dog

There are a great quantity of commercial foods and treats marketed for dogs, and not all are recommended as part of a balanced, healthy diet.

There is some debate as to whether domestic dogs should be classified as omnivores or carnivores, by diet. The classification in the Order Carnivora does not necessarily mean that a dog's diet must be restricted to meat; unlike an obligate carnivore, such as the cat family with its shorter small intestine, a dog is neither dependent on meat-specific protein nor a very high level of protein in order to fulfill its basic dietary requirements.

Dogs are able to healthily digest a variety of foods including vegetables and grains, and in fact dogs can consume a large proportion of these in their diet. Wild canines not only eat available plants to obtain essential amino acids, but also obtain nutrients from vegetable matter from the stomach and intestinal contents of their herbivorous prey, which they usually consume.

Domestic dogs can survive healthily on a reasonable and carefully designed vegetarian diet, particularly if eggs and milk products are included. Some sources suggest that a dog fed on a strict vegetarian diet without L-carnitine may develop dilated cardiomyopathy, however, L-carnitine is found in many nuts, seeds, beans, vegetables, fruits and whole grains. In the wild, dogs can survive on a vegetarian diet when animal prey is not available.

Observation of extremely stressful conditions such as the Iditarod Trail Sled Dog Race, and scientific studies of similar conditions has shown that high-protein (approximately 40 per cent) diets including meat help prevent damage to muscle tissue in dogs and some other mammals. This level of protein corresponds to the percentage of protein found in the wild dog's diet when prey is abundant; higher levels of protein seem to confer no added benefit.

Dogs frequently eat grass, which is a harmless activity. Explanations abound, but rationales such as that it neutralizes acid, or that dogs eat grass to induce vomiting to remove unwanted substances from their stomachs, are at best educated guesses. Dogs do vomit more readily than humans, as part of their typical feeding behaviour of gulping down food then regurgitating indigestible material such as bones and fur.

This behaviour is typical of pack feeding in the wild, where the most important thing is to get as much of the kill as possible before others consume it all. Individual domestic dogs, however, may be very "picky" eaters, in the absence of this social pressure. Dogs may also appear to eat grass when they are just running the blades through their mouth to gather information. Their sense of smell and taste may act together to detect if other animals have walked through their area or urinated on the grass.

DANGEROUS SUBSTANCES

Human food

Some foods commonly enjoyed by humans are dangerous to dogs, including chocolate (Theobromine poisoning), onions, grapes and raisins, some types of gum, certain sweeteners and Macadamia nuts. The only known dangerous substance in chocolate is cocoa, so the danger of white chocolate is uncertain. The acute danger from grapes and raisins was discovered around 2000, and has slowly been publicized since then. The cause is not known. Small quantities will induce acute renal failure. Sultanas and currants may also be dangerous. Cooked bones are dangerous for dogs, because the heat of cooking changes their chemical and physical properties so that they cannot be chewed properly. As a result they may splinter into jagged shards that resist digestion. Alcoholic beverages pose comparable hazards to dogs as they do to humans, but due to low body weight and lack of alcohol tolerance they are toxic in much smaller portions.

Plants

Plants such as caladium, dieffenbachia and philodendron will cause throat irritations that will burn the throat going down as well as coming up. Hops are particularly dangerous and even small quantities can lead to malignant hyperthermia. Amaryllis, daffodil, english ivy, iris, and tulip (especially the bulbs) cause gastric irritation and sometimes central nervous system excitement followed by coma, and, in severe cases, even death. Ingesting foxglove, lily of the valley, larkspur and oleander can be life threatening because the cardiovascular system is affected. Yew is very dangerous because it affects the nervous system. Immediate veterinary treatment is required for dogs that ingest these.

Household Poisons

Many household cleaners such as ammonia, bleach, disinfectants, drain cleaner, soaps, detergents, and other cleaners, mothballs and matches are dangerous to dogs, as are cosmetics such as deodorants, hair colouring, nail polish and remover, home permanent lotion, and suntan lotion. Dogs find some poisons attractive, such as antifreeze (automotive coolant), slug and snail bait, insect bait, and rodent poisons. Antifreeze is insidious to dogs, either puddled or even partly cleaned residue, because of its sweet taste. A dog may pick up antifreeze on its fur and then lick it off.

Animal feces

Dogs occasionally eat their own feces, or the feces of other dogs and other species if available, such as cats, deer, cows, or horses. This is known as coprophagia. Some dogs develop preferences for one type over another. There is no definitive reason known, although boredom, hunger, and nutritional needs have been suggested. Eating cat feces is common, possibly because of the high protein content of cat food. Dogs eating cat feces from a litter box may lead to to Toxoplasmosis. Dogs seem to have different preferences in relation to eating feces. Some are attracted to the stools of deer, cows, or horses.

Other risks

Human medications may be toxic to dogs, for example paracetamol/acetaminophen (Tylenol). Zinc toxicity, mostly in the form of the ingestion of US pennies minted after 1982, is commonly fatal in dogs where it causes a severe hemolytic anemia.

COW DIET

Corn has been a staple ingredient in lactating dairy cow rations for a hundred years. However, many dairy farms import corn to feed to their dairy cows. The price of this imported corn has been fairly stable for a number of years.

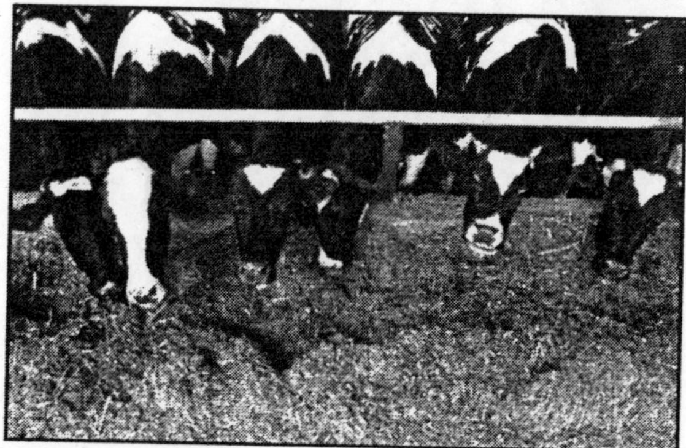

Fig. Feeding Dairy Cow

The government is trying to reduce dependence on foreign oil by supporting efforts to produce fuel (ethanol) from renewable resources like corn or cellulose. There is widespread public support for incorporating ethanol into fuelburning vehicles (gasoline and diesel) because ethanol addition results in greater combustion of these fuels and is nontoxic and biodegradable in the water and the soil.

The Congress passed legislation called a renewable fuels standard (RFS) that will at least double the use of ethanol and biodiesel by the year 2012. The number of plants producing ethanol from corn is projected to increase dramatically.

This growth in ethanol production has reduced the amount of corn available for livestock feed and concurrently increased its market price. Increased corn prices have resulted in increased feed costs. While higher milk prices may compensate for ration cost increases, partially replacing corn with other less expensive feedstuffs may be required over the longer term.

ALTERNATE RATION STRATEGIES

Other Grain Sources of Dietary Starch

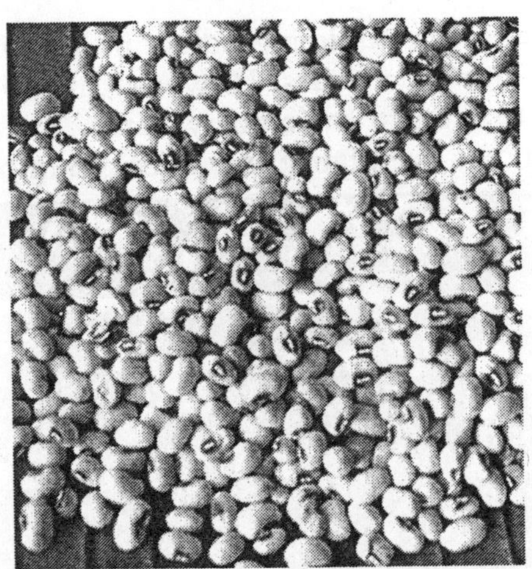

Fig. Grain Diet for cow

Grains, like corn, are an excellent source of starch which is highly fermentable by ruminal microorganisms. The propionic acid produced by starch-fermenting bacteria is converted to glucose by the cow's liver; this glucose is used to make milk. In addition, the bacteria provide about 50 to 60 per cent of the protein needs of the cow as they are washed out of the rumen and are digested in the abomasum and small intestine. To optimize milk production, starch should make up 24 to 26 per cent of the dietary dry matter. Barley and wheat are rich sources of dietary starch. Shifting cow diets between corn and barley or wheat needs to be done slowly.

The starch in barley and wheat is more rapidly available than that in corn so quick dietary changes can result in digestive upsets and lowered ruminal pH. Wheat flour can sometimes be bought for less than corn, but it is very dusty and potentially explosive so it is often avoided by mills. Field reports suggest that flour might 'paste up" in the rumen, so it is not a popular feed ingredient. Hominy contains less starch but more protein, fibre, and fat compared to corn, however their energy density is similar.

Replacing all of the corn with hominy will reduce the dietary starch concentration about 3 percentage units. Dietary costs would be expected to be reduced by replacing corn with hominy. If no milk is lost, then profit is improved. Experiments comparing performance of cows fed ground corn versus hominy could not be located. However, many Florida dairies feed hominy successfully. Even replacing half the corn with hominy can be a reasonable strategy. Because hominy is higher in fat and phosphorus than corn, care should be taken to avoid overfeeding these nutrients.

Low Starch Feedstuffs as Possible Substitutes for Corn

Because grain sources rich in starch, such as barley or wheat, may not be economically available year-round, other commodity feeds must be considered.

Ingredients with lower prices than corn should be considered as partial replacements for corn. Most common feedstuffs contain quite a bit less starch than corn. The best starch sources after corn include corn silage at 30 per cent, wheat midds at 26 per cent, wheat bran at 23 per cent, rice bran at 19 per cent, and corn gluten feed at 16 per cent (DM basis). All other feedstuffs are less than 10 per cent starch. Replacing some of the corn with these feeds will reduce dietary starch to less than 25 per cent which is a common, US ration target. How far can dietary starch be reduced without significantly affecting milk production?

Wheat Midds

Wheat midds contain 26 per cent starch and 18 per cent protein. Price can be substantially lower than corn at the right time of the year. Wheat midds have not been evaluated as a substitute for corn in many experiments. In a recent study, wheat midds were fed at about 7.5 per cent of the diet, replacing a combination of corn and soybean meal.

Corn was reduced in the diet from 34.1 to 28.9 per cent. Cows fed wheat midds tended to eat less feed dry matter but milk production and milk composition were not affected. This reduced feed intake may have been because wheat midds have a high water-holding capacity, thus increasing gut fill with fibre. Cows fed wheat midds appeared to have looser manure than those fed more corn and soybean meal.

In a second study, wheat midds were fed at 0 or 22.4 per cent of the diet, replacing 35 per cent of the ground corn and 30 per cent of the soybean meal. Intake of feed dry matter, production of milk, and milk composition were not different between the two groups of cows which averaged 150 days in milk at the start of the study. However the digestibility of dry matter and neutral detergent fibre were lower for cows fed wheat midds. Therefore wheat midds do not appear to be an effective feed replacement for ground corn except for lower producing cows.

Corn Feed

Corn gluten feed (CGF) is a byproduct of the manufacture of corn sweeteners, corn starch, corn syrup, and corn oil using the wet milling process. The corn starch is used to make ethanol. The CGF consists of the corn bran and a steep liquor (fermented nutrients extracted from water used to soak corn grain) mixed in approximately a 2:1 ratio. CGF is sold in both wet and dry forms. It contains 16 per cent starch, 36.1 per cent NDF, and 23.5 per cent protein, the protein being highly degradable in the rumen.

Pricing is substantially lower than corn. CGF may serve as a concentrate, replacing only the corn and soybean meal, or as both a concentrate and a fibre source, replacing both concentrate and traditional forages. CGF generally accounted for 10 to 45 per cent of the diet, although some studies went higher. When CGF was fed at about 20 per cent of ration DM, milk production was decreased statistically in 1 study, increased in 1 study, and remained unchanged in 9 other studies. Cows in these studies were milking between 50 and 90 pounds per day.

Increasing the CGF to 30, 40 or even 57 per cent of the diet did not reduce milk in any study with the exception of Staples et al. In two studies, in which CGF was fed between 38 and 40 per cent of the diet replacing both forage and concentrate starting at calving, average milk yield was increased significantly by feeding the corn gluten feed.

As more CGF replaced more corn, the dietary starch concentrations dropped, going as low as 15 per cent in some cases. In spite of lowered starch intake, milk yield did not drop significantly.

The bulk of these studies indicate that dietary starch could be reduced by replacing some corn and protein meals with the digestible fibre found in CGF.

Dropping dietary starch from 26 to 21 per cent may be an acceptable compromise. Sample diets were formulated to include CGF at 0 per cent, 10 per cent, and 20 per cent of the diet; starch was reduced concurrently from 25.9 to 23.5 per cent to 20.9 per cent in these rations. As CGF increases in diet, the proportion of extruded soy meal increased to keep the ruminally undegradable protein constant.

Degradable protein sources had to be reduced to keep the dietary crude protein from exceeding 17 per cent. Whether this approach will maintain milk production is not known. Milk and feed intake will be maintained when CGF is fed at 20 per cent of dietary DM. But feeding CGF at 10 per cent of the diet may be a preferred approach initially to "play it safe." Some signs that may indicate that the dietary starch has gotten too low include; dropped milk production, stiffer manure, increases in milk urea nitrogen, and loss of body condition.

Another concern is that drying CGF can reduce the digestibility of the protein if the drying temperature is too high.

This is determined by analyzing CGF for acid detergent insoluble protein (ADIN). Bernard et al.reported that dried CGF had higher concentrations of ADIN than wet CGF. In recent years, high ADIN may not be as big of a problem in CGF based upon analyses reported by Dairy One. The ADIN values were less than 5 per cent of the nitrogen in the majority of samples; ADIN is usually not considered a problem until it reaches 10 per cent of the total nitrogen in the feed.

Commodities need to have some consistent level of nutrient density from delivery to delivery in order to keep the daily ration nutrients consistent for the cows. Dairy One lists on their web site the normal range and standard deviation of the nutrients of most of the feeds they have analysed over the past 6 years.

Corn has an average starch value of 70.6 per cent. The standard deviation is 5.1 per cent. This means that two-thirds of the samples that were analysed ranged between 65.5 per cent and 75.7 per cent which is 5.1 per cent units added to or subtracted from the mean of 70.6 per cent. This also means that one-third of the samples analysed were outside this range. This is a fairly narrow range compared to byproduct feeds. Starch in CGF samples has a typical range of 8.6 per cent to 24.0 per cent with a mean of 16.3 per cent.

This large variation is likely due to the fact that CGF production is not standardized across mills. Likewise, starch in hominy typically ranges between 42.9 per cent and 63.9 per cent with a mean of 53.4 per cent. By feeding these byproducts in smaller amounts, the potential negative effect of nutrient variation on cow performance is reduced. When contracting for these commodities, an acceptable range in variation between loads should be agreed upon ahead of time. Loads delivered outside this agreed-upon-range would then be refused.

Dried Distillers Grains Plus Solubles (DDGS)

Dry corn put through the dry-milling process will produce ethanol, carbon dioxide, and DDGS. Each 56-pound bushel of corn processed through the dry milling process results in 2.85

gallons of ethanol, 18 pounds of carbon dioxide, and 18 pounds of DDGS. Plants using the dry milling process are less expensive to build than the plants using the wet milling process, thus about 75 per cent of the ethanol produced from corn comes from dry milling.

The production of DDGS in the US increased tenfold between the years 1980 and 2000, increasing from 320,000 to 3.5 million metric tons (1 metric ton = 2205 pounds). Production doubled again between 2000 and 2004 to over 7.3 million metric tons. Every dairy cow in the U.S. would need to consume 7.3 pounds per day of DDGS over a 305-day lactation in order to use up this supply, but of course DDGS is also fed to other livestock and is exported.

During the production of ethanol from corn, a syrup product and a cake product are produced. These products are blended together in different proportions to form DDGS. Depending on the plant, the DDGS may be a mixture of syrup to cake ranging in proportion from 35:65 to 55:45. Because of the variation in the ratio of syrup to cake used by different plants to form DDGS, nutrient concentrations will vary from one plant to another.

However the variation looks to be less than that of CGF. Although DDGS is very low in starch, it is an excellent source of protein (30.3 per cent) and fat (13 per cent) and therefore has an energy density very similar to corn. In addition, the ethanol-making process increases the digestibility of the fibre. Unlike CGF, DDGS is a very good source of ruminally undegradable protein (RUP) but if the temperature of the drying process is too high, the protein may be indigestible.

Purchasers of DDGS should analyse for ADIN regularly. Kalscheur et al. reviewed 24 experiments in which 98 comparisons were made between cows fed diets containing DDGS and those not fed DDGS. Cows fed DDGS at up to 30 per cent of the ration produced as much milk as those not fed any DDGS (about 73 lb/day). In spite of decreasing starch content, milk production was maintained. In a study conducted at the University of Florida, whiskey DDGS were fed at 0 per cent or 20 per cent of a 55 per cent concentrate:45

per cent forage diet. The forage was all corn silage in one set of diets and 50 per cent corn silage:50 per cent rhizome peanut silage in another set of diets. The DDGS replaced around 40 per cent of the corn and soybean meal. Milk production was increased from 59.0 to 60.7 pounds per day without changing milk fat test.

The effect of DDGS was the same regardless of whether the forage was totally corn silage or an equal mixture of corn silage and rhizome peanut silage. However, a maximum feeding level of DDGS might be 15 per cent in order to prevent the overfeeding of protein, RUP, unsaturated fat, and phosphorus. Increased corn oil in the DDGS can also lead to decreasing milk fat, so fat content of DDGS should be monitored regularly.

Feeding DDGS at 20 per cent of the diet will increase dietary fat by 2.6 per cent. This will likely be a concern if the diet contains other supplemental fats. Dietary fat should be kept below 6 per cent. The feeding of one pound of DDGS can replace about 0.6 pounds of corn and 0.4 pounds of soybean meal.

Soybean Hulls (SBH)

During the processing of soybeans for oil and meal, the hulls are separated and ground. The resulting soybean hulls consist largely of the outer covering of the soybean so they are high in fibre and contain moderate amounts of protein but very little starch. Protein concentration will depend upon how well the hulls are cleaned. Positive characteristics include a high content of lysine, a low content of phosphorus, and a highly digestible fibre. Fat content can vary widely.

The availability of SBH is likely to increase in coming years as more acres are planted to soybeans in order to use soybean oil for biodiesel production. In 13 separate experiments published between 1976 and 2002, SBH (fed at up to 20 per cent of the dietary DM) successfully replaced ground corn or high moisture corn in rations for lactating cows. In most of these studies, the dietary starch levels were probably greater than what is recommended today, based upon the proportion of corn in the diets fed in these studies. Therefore the replacement of corn with SBH still left enough starch to support adequate intake and milk production.

One study fed a more conservative amount of corn in the control diet and deserves further attention here. The control diet was 23 per cent high moisture corn, 26 per cent corn silage, and 26 per cent alfalfa silage. Adding SBH to the diet at 14 per cent of the dietary DM reduced the corn to 9 per cent of the diet. This dropped the starch from roughly about 25 per cent to 15 per cent, calculated from average values. Diets were fed starting at 8 days fresh.

Lactating cows ate more DM when offered the ration containing SBH but milk production was not changed. Lactating heifers fed SBH ate the same amount of feed and produced the same amount of milk as those not fed SBH. Concentrations of milk fat and protein were unchanged. Replacing 60 per cent of the corn with SBH, so that SBH made up 14 per cent of the ration, was effective to support high milk production in early lactation.

Even though dietary NDF increases when SBH replace corn, feed intake has not been decreased. This is in contrast with the well-documented fact that as traditional forage replaces concentrate in the diet, concentration of dietary NDF increases and feed intake decreases. However the NDF in nonforage fibre byproducts like SBH does not have the same physical characteristics as the NDF in traditional, properly chopped forage.

The fibre in SBH is highly digestible, very short and has a specific gravity that allows it to move out of the rumen quickly so that SBH fibre does not have the same rumen fill as forage fibre at similar NDF concentrations. In order to use SBH most efficiently, the diet should contain sufficient "effective" fibre from traditional forages.

Corn Silage

Corn silage hybrids differ in the proportion of grain in the total crop. Selecting corn silage hybrids that contain more starch will reduce the amount of ground corn needed. In a test of 55 corn silage hybrids grown in Gainesville in 2006, starch concentration ranged from 22 per cent to 35 per cent of silage dry matter, with an average of 29.3 per cent.

Selecting a corn silage hybrid with high levels of starch and digestible fibre, while maintaining high, could be a good strategy to reduce corn costs in the ration. How much could be saved? If a corn silage hybrid had 33 per cent starch instead of 30 per cent, and corn silage was fed at 33 per cent of the ration dry matter, dietary ground corn could be reduced from 18 per cent to 16.5 per cent, which is about 1 lb/day less ground corn. The cost savings would depend upon the relative price of the feedstuff(s) used.

Corn silage contains much more starch than other forages fed in Florida. Feeding more corn silage in the ration and less sorghum silage, cottonseed hulls, or bermudagrass will increase the starch in the diet and allow for less ground corn to be fed. If corn silage inventory allows, increasing the corn silage from 33 to 38 per cent of the diet DM by replacing another forage like sorghum silage, will allow ground corn to be reduced by 1.5 percentage units.

Glycerol

Glycerol is a byproduct made as plant and animal fats are processed to make diesel fuels. Diesel fuel produced from fat burns cleaner, as there is no soot or particulate matter produced. Starting with animal fat to make diesel fuel is more profitable than starting with vegetable oil because animal fats are cheaper. However, diesel made from animal fat may not work as well in colder climates because it "clouds up." This process is expanding worldwide and therefore the supply of glycerol in the future is likely to increase. Ten pounds of glycerol result from every 100 pounds of biodiesel produced.

The purity of this byproduct can vary widely. The more impure the product, the more water, methanol, phosphorus, and potassium it contains. A product with these contaminants is labeled glycerin. The glycerin fed in a German study contained 2.2 per cent potassium and up to 2.4 per cent phosphorus. Methanol is present due to its use in the manufacture of biodiesel. Although ruminal bacteria can detoxify methanol, it can be problematic if present in large quantities. According to the FDA, glycerin is considered a substance that is GRAS (Generally Recognized as Safe) for general purpose use in animal feed, unless methanol is present at concentrations exceeding 150 ppm. The energy content of glycerol is similar to corn when fed in high starch diets. Dietary glycerol would be converted mainly to propionate and butyrate by ruminal bacteria. As a feed ingredient, it could substitute for corn or molasses.

Little research has been done regarding the feeding of glycerol to dairy cows. Lactating dairy cows fed glycerol (1.3 per cent methanol) at either 0 per cent, 2.7 per cent, or 5.3 per cent of dietary dry matter ate the same amount of feed and produced the same amount of milk. Milk composition was unchanged with the exception that milk urea nitrogen concentrations were lower in cows fed glycerol.

Efficiency of fat-corrected milk production was improved from 1.46 to 1.59 and 1.60 lb of FCM yield per lb of feed dry matter intake. Interestingly, animals of other species consumed more water when they were fed glycerol. This may have a benefit to dairy cows managed under heat stress conditions. German researchers fed glycerol up to 10 per cent of ration DM successfully. Glycerol appears to be a good pelleting agent when added at 5 per cent.

Future Byproducts from new Technologies to improve Ethanol Production

As the ethanol manufacturing industry works at improving the efficiency of conversion of corn to ethanol, different byproducts will become available. Applegate et al. lists the following potential corn byproducts.

- Called the "quick germ quick fibre method," an enzyme is added to the water used to soak the ground corn, causing the germ and fibre to float before the fermentation process begins. The product from this process contains 28 per cent protein, 5 per cent fat, and 25 per cent NDF.

- Collecting the pericarp fibre and germ prior to fermentation by modifying the dry grinding process (drum degerminator) results in a product that is 24 per cent protein, 8-9 per cent fat, and 28 per cent NDF.
- Removing the fibre by sieving and air aspiration results in a product that is 40+ per cent protein, 15 per cent fat, and 20 per cent NDF.
- Modifying the yeasts used to ferment the sugar to ethanol could allow for an increased concentration of lysine in DDGS, thus giving DDGS a more favourable amino acid profile.

As each mill adopts what they consider the best ethanol-producing technology, the feeding industry will be faced with a variety of byproducts on the market which will need to be properly identified prior to purchase.

With the increased price for corn due to demand for ethanol, farmers will be planting more of their acres to corn. This will reduce the number of acres committed to other crops, such as cottonseed. This shift will likely have a large impact on the market price of a number of feed commodities. The availability and price of each commodity will need to be evaluated for optimal pricing. Some acceptable, alternative feeds may allow some reduction of corn grain in the diet of lactating dairy cows.

FEEDING GOATS

Feeds for goats can be divided into several different categories: forages, grains, protein supplements, minerals and water. Depending on what levels of each category that is fed. It will be found that goats will gain about.25 to.5 a pound each day.

Goats will readily eat a variety of forages. These include pasture, hay, haylage, and brush. Any species of forage is acceptable for goats, although be careful of feeding a lot of alfalfa to wethers and billies because the higher calcium levels can lead to urinary calculi or kidney stones. Goats are very useful in many operations for cleaning up unwanted brushy areas. Most brushy areas will only be able to survive about 2 years with intensive defoliation. Forages are an important part of a ruminant's ration because the high fibre is necessary to keep the digestive system healthy. Grains provide the energy portion of a ration for goats. A variety of grains are available, with corn, oats, wheat and barley being the most widely used. Limit the amount of wheat in the ration to no more than 2 per cent to prevent any digestive problems. When starting goats on a feedlot ration, be sure to gradually introduce them to grain.

Feeding high levels of grain suddenly can cause bloating and overeating disease. Disease can be prevented by vaccinating with type C and D perfringens. This is often available in one vaccine, along with tetanus. Any male goats that are castrated should receive a dose of tetanus vaccine. Castration is a personal consideration as many ethnic groups prefer to purchase intact males.

Protein Supplements

Market goats should be fed a grain ration that runs between 14 per cent and 18 per cent protein. To reach these protein levels, we need to include some sort of protein supplement. Typical supplements will include soybean meal, roasted soybeans, cottonseed, brewers or distiller's grains, or flour mill by-products. Beware of using any dairy protein supplements because of the amount of copper in the supplements. Many nutritionists still disagree over the amount of copper required in a goat ration, but care should still be given to overfeeding this nutrient.

Minerals

One of the best ways to provide minerals to a market goat is through a commercially mixed salt and mineral mix. Be sure to purchase a mix formulated specifically for goats. Allow goat's free access to a mineral feeder that contains the mineral mix at all times. Minerals are especially important for helping to ensure that goats remain healthy. These mineral mixes will often include some of the essential vitamins for goats as well.

Water

Water is often one of the most overlooked aspects of livestock feeding operations. Clean, fresh water should be available at all times for all species of livestock. Animals that have adequate amounts of water are more likely to stay healthy as well as have a faster growth rate. Goats will often be able to supply all of their water needs through dew and lush pasture. However, it is still in their best interest to have a supply of water available to them at all times.

OTHER FEED ADDITIVES

For herds that are prone to urinary calculi, ammonium chloride can be added to prevent the disease. Another common practice is to add a coccidiostat to the ration to prevent as well as control coccidiosis. Common additives used to prevent coccidiosis include Rumensin, Bovatec or Deccox (decoquinate). Lastly, no matter what the ration, be sure to provide enough feeder space for all the goats to eat. Plan for at least 1 foot of feeder space for each goat. And, don't forget to clean feeders and waterers on a regular basis.

Sound feeding practices and good housing facilities result in optimum growth and high milk production and contribute to the good health and comfort of goats.

When feeding goats, keep these objectives must be in mind:

- Feed a young animal enough energy for growth, and feed a mature animal enough energy to maintain a fairly constant body weight;
- Provide enough protein, minerals and vitamins in a balanced feeding programme to maintain a healthy animal; and
- Offer does enough extra food during gestation and lactation for fetus development and milk production.

Optimum growth, good health and high milk production are the results of sound feeding practices. Dairy goats are not unique in their body requirements; they will respond to good nutritional practices. Digestible fibre is especially important in dairy goat diets. Too much grain in relation to forage does not foster good ruminant action and is a costly feeding practice. When feeding, keep minerals and trace mineral salt separate. Always feed them separately.

Feed hay in a rack that will not permit wasting. One recommended type of feeder is a keyhole feeder. Do not overlook forage testing as an economical way to feed the correct ration to herd.

Feeding Kids and Yearlings

Kids are born with no natural protection from disease. The first milk (colostrum) from the mother offers protection and gets the digestive system working. To be most effective, it must be fed before disease-producing organisms enter the mouth and digestive tract. Wash the fresh doe's udders and teats with warm water.

Hand milk half a cup of colostrum and feed it to the kid within 15 minutes of birth. This is the best way to ensure that the newborn receives some milk and to provide it with the most protection from organisms present on the skin of the doe. Complete the first milking and store the colostrum for later feedings if hand feed is elected. Otherwise, permit the kid to nurse at its convenience following the first hand feeding.

Clean the feeding utensils immediately after each use. The same cleaning procedures should be followed for washing milk-handling equipment. Milk replacer may be fed from the fourth day; it should contain at least 20 percent protein, 20 percent fat and be free of vegetable products. A lamb or high-quality calf milk replacer is recommended. Provide hay and grain at one to two weeks of age.

Wean from milk when grain intake reaches 1/4-pound daily and kids are readily consuming hay. Make sure the solution is thoroughly mixed. Mix a fresh mixture daily and feed in place of milk. Feed as soon as diarrhea is noticed. Use for 1-1/2 or 2 days, then return to the regular milk diet. After four to six months of age, the kids may be fed a ration similar to that of the milking herd. Good hay and 1/2 pound of grain per day should provide an ample growth rate. Poor hay may require 1 to 1-1/2 pounds of grain daily.

Feeding the Milking Herd

If milk production is important, feed maximum amounts of high quality hay balanced with a grain ration containing enough protein, minerals and vitamins to support production and animal health. Grass or legume hays are equally acceptable. As the percentage of legumes is increased, the need for protein in the grain mix is reduced.

To determine the amount of grain to feed, consider level of milk production, amount and quality of forages consumed, appetite and state of fleshing. Thin, high-producing does should have access to all the hay they can eat plus grain to the limit of their appetite. Does in mid-lactation that are in good flesh should have all the hay they will eat plus 1 pound of grain for each 3 pounds milk produced. Late lactation does may not need more than 1 pound of grain for each 5 pounds of milk.

Feed a grain ration formulated for a milk-producing ruminant (dairy cows). Rolled or cracked grain is more palatable than ground grain. Because of palatability problems, urea is not recommended. Some commercial cow feeds may contain byproduct ingredients unpalatable to goats. Wet molasses is more palatable than dry molasses. Beer or citrus pulp is a valuable source of fibre, especially if the available hay is of low quality.

If the doe is not thin, reduce the amount of grain to 1/2 to 1 pound per day. Feed her all the forage she will eat. Hay fed during the dry period may be of lower quality, but if so, the grain ration should contain additional protein. Browse, leaves and weeds are often useful to recondition the stomach. If the dry ration differs from the milking ration, be sure to change to the milking forage and grain ration two weeks before the doe freshens. Most bucks do not need more than a pound of grain per day plus forages. Don't let them grow fat. Adjust grain upward or downward accordingly. Always feed full forage.

FEEDING AND NUTRITION OF PIG

Feeding guinea pig is a fairly simple manner, though there

are a few special needs that we should be aware of. Guinea pigs are strict vegetarians, and in addition to their pellets, they will eat fruits and vegetables, bread, and will even nibble on vegetarian dog biscuits.

Before getting in to the details, it is important to point out that guinea pigs like a routine, predictable life. Sudden changes in their diet can cause stress, so be careful. If the brands of pellets is changed, gradually by adding a few of the new ones to their old pellets, and slowly switching the mixture over. Feeding excessive amounts of fruits and vegetables at one time can cause diarrhea, particularly if new foods are introduced.

All guinea pigs need water to survive. Though they can obtain a large portion of their water from fresh fruits, vegetables and greens, they will still require water from a water bottle to stay healthy. This water should be changed daily, and the water bottles themselves washed periodically to keep them clean. To prevent algae growth, make sure that the sun does not directly shine on the water bottle for long periods of time.

If there is arrangement of tap water bottled water or a water filter system should be considered. Distilled water is not recommended for regular drinking, as it can disturb the osmotic pressure in the body cells, which can potentially lead to osmotic shock.

Be aware that some guinea pigs like to "play" with their water bottle, leaking out large amounts of water by holding the steel ball up in the tube. Others like to try and blow water back up into the bottle, which can contaminate the entire supply.

Hay is the mainstay of every guinea pig's diet. Though guinea pig pellets do contain hay, it is not in sufficient quantity to keep guinea pig healthy. Guinea pig must have a fresh supply of hay every day in order to keep its digestive system regular, and as a general rule.

Timothy hay is the best type of hay to feed, though any grass hay will do. If grass hay is not available, a legume hay can be fed, such as alfalfa, though in general this should be avoided as much as possible. Legume hays are high in calcium, and this can lead to bladder stones (uroliths) in some animals.

Most pet stores carry dried timothy hay in large and small bags, but it is far better to purchase hay fresh from a feed and garden store, or directly from a farmer. Buying hay by the bale is especially economical, as a bale of hay will literally last for months, and will stay fresh as long as it is stored properly. Some tips on hay storage can be found here.

Guinea Pig pellets

Guinea pig pellets will provide guinea pig with the proper balance of vitamins (save for Vitamin C), minerals and other nutrients. Although it's not necessary to feed pellets to guinea pigs, it is certainly recommended that they be primary feed, after hay. Guinea pig pellets are, in particular, a prime source of protein; obtaining the necessary amounts of this and other nutrients will require careful dietary planning if pellets are not chosen.

As a general rule of thumb, adult guinea pigs will eat between one and two ounces of pellets each day. More active animals will eat less, and animals without much stimulation will eat more out of boredom. Nursing and pregnant sows may demand a little more than this, and animals that are given plenty of hay and some fresh vegetables each day might eat a little less. It will be easy to tell if they are fed too much or too little: if there are leftover pellets. If the bowl is empty and they seem to be foraging for food, then they aren't fed enough.

Try to feed at the same hour each day, as guinea pigs like a routine and predictable life. Remove any leftover pellets after an hour or so. Guinea pig pellets are a prime source of protein: a diet that is heavy on pellets will lead to a fat guinea pig. Hay is the only food that they should have access to 24 hours a day.

When choosing pellets, be sure to *avoid* the guinea pig "mixes" that contain nuts, seeds and dried fruits. These mixes are high in fats and oils, which can lead to excessive weight gain. Additionally, many of these mixes contain sunflower seeds in their shells. Guinea pigs should *never* be fed nuts or seeds that are still in their shells (peanuts, sunflower seeds, etc.): dozens of guinea pigs in the Pacific Northwest alone die each year from choking on these shell fragments.

One thing that should be noted before we move on: guinea pigs should be fed guinea pig pellets, not rabbit pellets or pellets for another species of animal. Guinea pig pellets are nutritionally balanced for guinea pigs, and feeding them pellets for other animals can result in serious health problems.

Though some people may tell that their guinea pigs survive well on rabbit pellets, for instance, it is not trusted that all rabbit food is safe for guinea pigs. Their particular brand may work for guinea pigs, but another brand may lack necessary vitamins or minerals, or have them in insufficient or excessive quantities.

There is no regulation in the pet food industry, so pellets and feeds vary considerably between manufacturers. Don't play Russian roulette with cavies: only feed them pellets that are explicitly and *exclusively* for guinea pigs.

It is *extremely important* that guinea pigs receive enough vitamin C each day to prevent scurvy. Guinea pigs cannot manufacture or store vitamin C, so they must obtain it from their diet on a daily basis. Adult guinea pigs will require 10mg of vitamin C each day, and nursing and pregnant sows will require twice that amount (20mg). The caveat: vitamin C, also known as ascorbic acid, breaks down very quickly, so it must be supplied fresh. Although many pellet manufacturers will claim that their feed contains the required amount of vitamin C.

Vitamin C in pellets breaks down during storage, and after about 90 days, there won't be enough vitamin C in the feed to keep guinea pigs healthy. Also note that the food starts breaking down on the shelf, not when the bag of pellets are opened. Unless the manufacturer dates the bag, showing when the feed was packaged, we really have no idea how long pellets have been on the shelf at the local pet store.

Since pellets are generally an inadequate source of vitamin C, most owners will either feed sufficient quantities of fruits and vegetables rich in vitamin C each day, or provide vitamin

C in the form of supplements added to the guinea pigs' food or drinking water.

Vitamin supplements come in many forms: pre-packaged vitamin supplements for guinea pigs can be bought from pet store, or self grind up vitamin C tablets. In either case, most people prefer to add the vitamins to the animal's drinking water, as that is the only way to guarantee that it will be ingested daily. If the supplement routes are chosen, here are a few pointers:

- Add the appropriate amount of supplement to the amount of water that the guinea pig will drink in a day. Most water bottles work best if they are filled halfway or more, so end up wasting a lot of vitamins. Fortunately, they aren't very expensive. If guinea pig drinks 4 fluid ounces of water a day, and fill water bottle with 8 ounces, then need to add 20mg of vitamin C supplement. This will lead to 4 ounces of wasted water and 10 mg of wasted vitamin C.
- Vitamin C (ascorbic acid) breaks down very quickly in water, so need to add it on a daily basis.
- The chlorine in tap water can actually inactivate ascorbic acid. If vitamin supplements in water is opted, then use tap water that has been standing for at least 24 hours, or filtered tap water from a filter system that reduces chlorine content.

Being vegetarians, guinea pigs will eat many kinds of fruits, vegetables and fresh greens. And, many fruits and vegetables are sources of vitamin C, providing a natural way to meet guinea pig's daily requirement.

Calcium and Phosphorus totals for the given food amounts are presented as well. Although these are necessary minerals, and a part of every guinea pig's diet, they are getting them from their pellets, as well. The nutrients guinea pig is getting along with their vitamin C. Too much calcium can cause bladder sludge, a precursor to bladder stones. The proper balance of phosphorus, calcium and vitamin C prevents guinea pigs from needing vitamin D supplements.

Although most guinea pig pellets contain vitamin D as a

precaution, there's no guarantee that particular brand of feed does. In addition to providing vitamin C and variance in cavy's diet, fresh greens and fruits contain a significant amount of water. Feeding "wet foods" will aid nursing sows in lactating, and will reduce the amount of water that the average guinea pig will drink from the water bottle.

It is especially useful to take lettuce, green peppers and other watery greens on trips to provide moisture for guinea pigs while in the car, since water bottles will leak heavily as the bumps in the road rattle the ball in the drinking tube.

To reduce or completely eliminate pellets from guinea pig's diet, they can survive on water, hay and fresh fruits and vegetables. However, this will require very careful dietary planning on part, to make sure that they receive the necessary nutrients in the proper amounts. Also, be aware that many fresh greens are laxative in action, which means that run the risk of giving guinea pigs loose bowels, or even diarrhea, if the are fed too much at one time. If runny droppings are noticed immediately cut fresh greens out of their diet and feed dry foods until the feces returns to normal. Vegetables that are not laxative (such as carrots) may still be fed.

Guinea pigs will not eat what they don't like: some cavies have very discriminating tastes, while others will eat anything that put in front of them. Each pig has its own preferences, and it may take some time to figure out what he or she likes best. Given below is a list of foods that guinea pigs can/will eat. This list is neither comprehensive nor complete.

Apples, bananas, bread (slightly stale & crunchy, but not moldy), broccoli, carrot greens, carrots and baby carrots, celery (cut into small pieces first), cilantro, cucumber, dandelion greens, grass, green & red bell peppers, green leaf & romaine lettuce, kale, kiwi, mustard greens, oats, oranges, parsley, raspberries, spinach, tomatoes.

When feeding "wild" greens, such as grass and dandelion greens, make sure they have not been sprayed with chemicals, or contaminated by droppings or urine from other animals, such as cats, dogs and birds. The dangers of pesticides are obvious, and feces can carry any number of parasites which can be transmitted to cavies eating contaminated greens. Even if dogs and cats are dewormed regularly, their feces can contain protozoa/bacteria which can cause debilitating diarrhea in a guinea pig.

Some foods to avoid are listed below:

- Long celery stalks
- Iceberg lettuce
- Any shelled nuts or seeds
- Raw beans
- Rhubarb

There is some confusion as to whether or not potato peelings are good or bad: some books indicate that they are poisonous to guinea pigs, while others say that they are okay in small amounts. The truth is that potatoes are *okay,* however, any *green* in a potato *is poisoinous.*

If potato peelings are given, make sure there are *no green spots* anywhere in the portions. Also, some people may recommend yogurt in small amounts, for it's bacteria-growing properties (to aid the digestive system). Instead, look into acidophilus powders or liquids: acidophilus is also a bacteria growing culture, and it';s likely to give better results since less of it needs to be fed.

There are several commercially available treats on the market that are aimed at guinea pigs. Berry flavoured "crunchies" and flavoured chew sticks are popular among some owners and guinea pigs, and are generally safe. Some owners also have experimented with vegetarian dog biscuits and dry cereals such as Cheerio's.

However, the guinea pig "treat sticks", which are also available commercially. These sticks are essentially seeds and nuts that are held together with honey. Most of the treat sticks on the market contain sunflower seeds that are still in their shells, which is a big no-no for guinea pigs due to the choking hazards.

FISH FEEDING

Providing fish with the right type of food in the right proportions is a very important task. This can be much more of a challenge in a saltwater tank than in a freshwater tank, because most marine fish are still wild-caught, and their natural diet can be difficult to maintain in captivity. With the right information, however, most marine fish will learn to eagerly anticipate their feeding time and will voraciously devour their food.

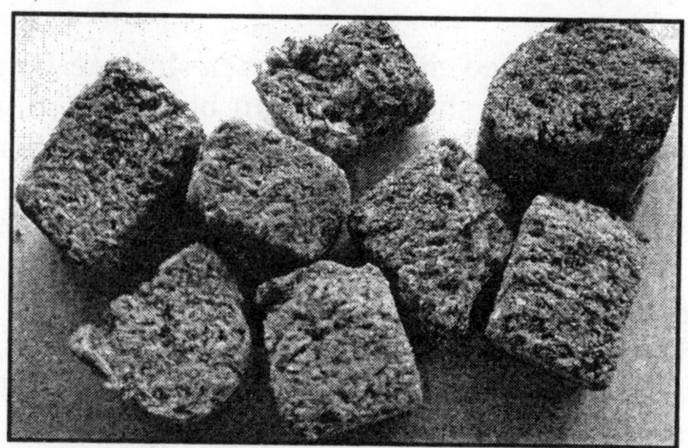

Fig. Fish Food

A good rule of thumb to follow is that fish should be fed no more than they can consume within a five minute period. Any food that is left behind after feeding time should be removed before it has a chance to begin decomposing. If it is found that fish are consuming the food in far shorter a time than five minutes and seem anxious for more, the amount that are fed must be increased.

On the other hand, if fish are healthy, but they are only consuming about half of what they are fed, probably need to start feeding less. Always keep in mind that much more harm can be done to fish by overfeeding than by underfeeding.

In the wild, reef fishes will browse for food throughout the day. Their natural habitat as closely as possible, it is recommended that fish must be fed several small meals every day. At the very least, feed two medium-sized meals per day, one in the morning and one at night.

Types of Fish Food

The kind of food to feed depends on the kind of fish are feeding: herbivore, carnivore, or omnivore.

Herbivores

It is common for fish that graze on algae in the wild to suffer in captivity because they don't receive the appropriate type of food to keep them healthy. Many of these fish are fed terrestrial greens like spinach and romaine lettuce, but these are not appropriate foods for these fish that are solely algae eaters.

They should be fed either dried or fresh algae. Dried algae is sold in paper-thin sheets that can be broken down into appropriate portion sizes, depending on the number of fish are feeding. Fresh algae can be obtained by placing a glass container, with one rock in aquarium, on a sunny windowsill. Wait for the rock to grow a nice layer of algae, and then place it back in the aquarium for fish to graze on.

Herbivorous fish can also be fed one of the frozen fish foods that is formulated especially for herbivores. This food should contain a variety of marine algae, vegetable matter, and seafood. Whether herbivorous fish are fed dried algae, fresh algae, or a frozen food formula, herbivorous eaters are grazers and should have food available to them at all times, unlike most other fish.

Carnivores

Meat-eating marine fish can enjoy a variety of fresh, frozen, freeze-dried, and live foods. Fresh foods suitable for fish include many seafood items, such as shrimp, scallops, mussels, clams, and some fish. If seafood is fed to fish, cut it into bite-sized pieces (or serve it whole to larger fish). Fresh seafood can be frozen and then thawed as needed.

Frozen foods are available from most fish shops and other sources. These offerings may include brine shrimp, bloodworms, and daphnia. They may be in the form of a slab that can be broken into smaller pieces or small, ready-to-go cubes. To feed frozen foods to carnivorous fish, thaw a small portion in aquarium water, and then drop it in the tank.

Several freeze-dried foods for carnivorous fish are readily available, such as plankton, krill, brine shrimp, and bloodworms. Freeze-dried foods are foods that have been completely dehydrated, yet they maintain most of their nutritional value. They have a relatively long shelf life, particularly when compared to fresh and frozen foods. Freeze-dried foods should be used as supplements for carnivorous fish. Live foods are almost always a favourite of fish. Adult brine shrimp, bloodworms, and Mysis shrimp are among the better choices. Earthworms are also a great live food choice because they come in all sizes, fish love them. Be sure to thoroughly rinse them before feeding them to fish.

Omnivores

The majority of marine fish are omnivorous, which means they need to eat both meat- and plant-based foods. One easy option for omnivorous eaters is commercial fish food, such as flakes or pellets. However, offering a varied diet will give healthier, more colourful fish. Try to feed fish two feedings a day of commercial fish food and one feeding of a meaty item, such as bloodworms or chopped fish. The food offered must be alternated in addition to commercial food to keep the fish from getting bored and to make sure all of their nutritional needs are met.

SHEEP DIET

Sheep are exclusively herbivorous mammals. Like all ruminants, sheep have a complex digestive system composed of four chambers that allows them to break down otherwise inedible cellulose from stems, leaves, and seed hulls in to complex carbohydrates.

When sheep graze, vegetation is chewed in to a mass called a bolus, which is then passed in to the first chamber: the rumen. The rumen is a 5-10 gallon (18.9-37.8 liter) organ which ferments feed via a symbiotic relationship with the millions of bacterium, protozoa, and yeasts which are collectively called flora.

The bolus is periodically regurgitated back in to the mouth as cud for additional chewing and salivation, this process usually takes around six hours. Cud chewing is an evolutionary adaptation that allows ruminants to graze more quickly in the morning, and then fully chew and digest feed later in the day. This is beneficial because grazing, which requires lowering the head, leaves sheep more vulnerable to predators, while cud chewing does not.

During fermentation, the rumen produces excess gas which must be expelled; disturbances of the organ, such as sudden changes in a sheep's diet, can cause potentially fatal conditions such as bloat. After fermentation in the rumen, feed passes in to the reticulum and the omasum; special feeds such as grains may bypass the rumen altogether.

Following the first three chambers, food moves in to the abomasum for final digestion before processing by the intestines. The abomasum is the only one of the three chambers directly equatable with the usual mammalian stomach, and is accordingly sometimes called the "true stomach".

Sheep follow a diurnal pattern of activity, beginning to feed at dawn and throughout the day until dusk, stopping sporadically to rest and chew their cud. Ideal pasture for sheep is not lawn-like grass, but an array of grasses, legumes and forbs. Types of land where sheep are raised vary widely, from pastures that are seeded and improved intentionally to rough, native lands. Common plants toxic to sheep are present in most of the world, and include (but are not limited to) oak and acorns, tomato, yew, rhubarb, potato, and rhododendron. Sheep also may perish from consuming man-made substances.

Sheep are largely grazing herbivores, unlike browsing animals such as goats and deer that prefer taller foliage. With a much narrower face, they can crop plants very close to the ground and can overgraze a pasture much faster than cattle. For this reason, many shepherds utilize some type of managed grazing, whereby a flock is rotated through multiple pastures, giving plants time to recover.

Paradoxically, sheep can be both the cause of and solution to one of the major ill effects of overgrazing: the spread of invasive plant species. By disturbing the natural make-up of pasture, sheep and other livestock can pave the way for invasive plants. But sheep also prefer to eat invasives such as cheatgrass, leafy spurge, kudzu and spotted knapweed over native species such as sagebrush—thereby making grazing sheep an effective measure in restoring native pastures.

Other than forage, the only other common staple feed for sheep is hay, most often during the winter months. The ability to survive solely on pasture (even without hay) varies with breed, but all sheep are capable of doing so. Also included in most sheep's diets are minerals, either in a trace mix or in licks.

Naturally, a constant source of potable water is also a fundamental requirement for sheep. The amount of water needed by sheep fluctuates with the season and the type and quality of the food they consume. When sheep feed on large amounts of new growth and there is precipitation (including dew, as sheep are dawn feeders), sheep need less water. When sheep are confined or are eating large amounts of cured hay, more water is typically needed. Sheep also require clean water, and may refuse to drink water that is covered in scum or algae.

COOLING PONDS FOR DAIRY CATTLE

Cattle have used water for cooling probably for as long as there have been cattle. The last survey done in Florida reported that 30 per cent of the dairies had cooling ponds. The reader should be aware that cooling ponds, if not maintained properly, could harbor infectious diseases such as Leptospirosis and many mastitis organisms. The water usage is very high to fill and keep full.

Environmental concerns that must be addressed are the run-off from ponds and ground seepage. Every state seems to have many regulations that must be addressed before building cooling ponds. The benefits of cooling ponds and some suggestions on building and maintaining them. It is the dairymen's responsibility to use them properly and to be aware that ponds can harbor diseases and the pond water must be dealt with according to state and local laws.

What is a cooling pond for dairy cattle? For this discussion they are a man made hole in the ground with a constant inflow of clean fresh water. Usually the ponds drain or overflow from the top. If a series of ponds is used, the overflow water may be run into a retention pond to be irrigated on crops or enter the waste management system. Cooling ponds may also be fed from springs or artesian wells. So cooling ponds for dairy cattle should have constant fresh water in and a constant outflow of water to some place for proper disposal.

Cement ponds may also be built. These may drain from the bottom and can be used to flush feed lanes or barns. Bottom draining will help remove some of the solids that have settled to the bottom of the pond. Care must be taken on the entrance and exit to cement ponds.

These may be very slippery if the cement is not cross-grooved. A stagnant pond without fresh water entering, a lagoon, a wallow, and a mud hole do not classify as a cooling pond for dairy cattle.

Site Selection

A site near the feed and drinking water, ideally with some form of shade for cows, is best. The idea is for cows to cool, leave the pond and goes eat and drink, lay down in the shade and then do it all over again. If cows do not have feed and drinking water near, they will stay in the pond and not eat and we have cool wrinkled cows that do not give much milk.

Cooling ponds should be located close to a water supply as fresh water needs to enter the ponds constantly. There must be a way to dispose of runoff water properly. This will vary by areas of the country.

Some slope from the ponds to the waste management area would be helpful, so pumps need not to be used. Cooling ponds should not be too far from the milking parlor as long walks in the sun increase heat stress. Exit lane sprinklers help make the long walk more comfortable.

Concrete Ponds

Concrete ponds will work and have been used but they are expensive to build. However, they are easier to maintain, as the entrances and exits do not have to be rebuilt. The finish of the concrete on exit and entrance slopes should be cross-grooved to prevent cows from falling. A 1:8 slope would be a safe slope if concrete ponds are constructed.

Sizing Cooling Ponds

There is no official listing for cooling pond size. If a holding area requires 15/ft^2 / cow and cows are driven into a pond and taken out as a group then 15/ft^2 / cow might be adequate. If 50/ft^2 / cow is recommended for most general animal space, then this might be the correct figure for a cooling pond.

This amount of space would allow cows to enter and exit the pond at all times when all cows were not using the pond at the same time. If 50/ft^2 / cow for a pond is used, then 5000/ ft^2 is then needed for the 100 cow group.

Pond Shapes and Depths

Using the sample of 5000/ft^2 /100 cows a pond could be 50' wide × 100' long, or a circle 80' in diameter (A= (Pi) r^2; A= 3.14 × 40 = 5024ft^2). If a 50' × 100' pond is used and the sides are fenced so the cows can only enter or exit at each end of the pond, the amount of dirt falling into the pond will be reduced. If a circular pond is made, cow carpet should be used to eliminate the problem of dirt falling in the pond. As cows can swim, pond depth is not a problem.

Deeper ponds may allow the settling of organic matter on the bottom of the pond. This organic matter may not be disturbed by cows walking through it as they will swim over the top of it. Preference should be given to depths of 3' or 4' as it seems to cool the cows and let them stand and walk in and out at will. While deep ponds allow cows to submerge, they do not seem to like to float too long so they go to where they can stand and may block cow traffic. A circular pond that is deep in the middle lets cows dunk themselves while others enter and exit the pond at will.

Water Usage

A 100 cow group with 50/ft^2 / cow could have a 50' wide × 100' long × 3' deep cooling pond (it may be 4' in the middle and slope in and out). A cooling pond 50' wide × 100' long × an average 3' deep=15000/ft^3. There are 7.48 gallons/ft^3, thus the pond requires 112,200 gallons of water.

The pond must be filled and then kept fresh with running water at all times while in use. A 1" pipe 300 ft. long and water pressure at 35psi will result in a flow rate of about 23.5 gpm. At this rate it would then take 80 hours to fill the pond initially.

The dairy water usage would then be 1,410 gph × 24 hours or 33,840 gallons of water per day. This fresh water must be pumped into the pond and there is going to be close to that amount of run off water that will exit the pond for disposal.

Water Run-off

Disposal of run-off water must be in accordance with whatever local, state, and federal laws that applies. Many dairies run the water into the waste management system, while others add it to retention ponds to be used for irrigation.

Shading over Ponds

Experience has led to discontinued use of shade over ponds as the cows never leave the ponds. Remember, the object of this exercise is to increase dry matter intake and cows will not eat much soaking in the pond.

Pond Maintenance

At least once a year, usually during the winter, the pond should be fenced and the water removed by pumping. The mud and manure on the bottom of the pond should be removed and the pond left empty for the sun to shine on it.

In the spring, the pond should be filled again and the fences removed. Some people just fence the pond in the winter, dig a new pond and fill in the old one with new pond's dirt.

Mycoplasma mastitis is often cultured in water from cooling ponds. This is a real problem if pulsators do not work well resulting in damaged teat ends. Many herds with mycoplasma positive ponds, have no mycoplasma in the bulk tank.

If the water is filthy, cows should not be permitted in the ponds and the ponds should be pumped dry. The sludge should be cleaned and the ponds filled with water again. Both the sludge and the water shoud be removed from cow areas.

Cooling Ponds to Reduce Body Temperature

In the summer of 1986, an experiment was conducted at a North Florida dairy that was using man-made cooling ponds. Ten early lactation Holstein cows were fitted with radio transmitters that transmitted inner ear temperatures every five minutes to a radio receiver and data logger.

Data were collected over a four-day period in mid-August. The cows' activities were also monitored during this time. Entering and exiting the ponds, eating, drinking and laying were recorded.

The cooling ponds lowered the cows' temperature by 1-2°F depending on the time of day they entered the cooling ponds. The average length per stay in the pond was 18 minutes for events from midnight to noon and 12 minutes per visit from noon to midnight. It was obvious that cooling ponds cooled cows.

Pond Water Quality

In 1987, samples were taken from a dairy's man-made earthen ponds. The ponds were sampled weekly from May 19,1987 to September 28, 1987. Six to ten ponds were sampled each week.

Total bacteria counts (TBC), varied greatly from week to week. This may have been due to no water entering the ponds. There did not seem to be any great increase in total bacteria counts or coliform counts as time progressed. The total bacteria count averaged 3,133,700 CFU/ml for all ponds for the 20 weeks. The coliform counts averaged 14,340 CFU/ml for the same period.

Cooling Ponds and Their Effect on Milk Quality

In a previous study on a dairy in Florida with man-made cooling ponds, it was reported that cows exposed to cooling ponds did not experience more clinical mastitis than cows that did not have access to cooling ponds. In fact, cows exposed to cooling ponds during the trial period were only half as likely to develop a case of clinical mastitis as cows not exposed to cooling ponds.

Clinical Mastitis Organisms

The same dairy had provided its clinical mastitis records for several years. The total number of clinical mastitis cases was high in the first quarter of the year and then declined sharply about the time hot weather came and the cows started using the ponds. The incidence stayed low, even in the last quarter of the year when the ponds were not in use. This can be explained many ways. The first quarter of the year was an extremely wet period.

The cows were quite dirty and the cow wash system was available to one-half of the herd. This may explain some of the variation, even though one-half of the herd had never had a cow wash. Another confounding variable was that this herd switched to Clorox for pre- post-teat dipping in April of that year. It had previously pre- and post-dipped with a Chlorhexidine product. From this it could be concluded that Clorox caused the reduction of clinical mastitis. However, there were no controls in this study, one could conclude nothing except that the ponds did not increase clinical mastitis.

This herd was on a lactation treatment study during the summer of 1987. A total of 40 cows were sampled and treated. There were no unusual organisms treated. These 40 cows were not all the cows treated for clinical mastitis during the period the cows had access to the ponds, but the results were encouraging.

Statewide Effects of Ponds on Milk Quality

Regulatory samples for all the herds in Florida were obtained from the Division of Dairy Industry for the year of 1987 and were analysed for the effects of no ponds, man-made ponds and natural ponds. The numbers presented are least squares estimates of Standard Plate Counts (SPC) and Direct Microscope Somatic Cell Counts (DMSCC) for each month. The data are not biased by different numbers of dairies with no ponds, natural, or man-made ponds. The data were analysed by herds whose milking cows had access to ponds as indicated on the survey.

The data indicated that milking cows with access to man-made cooling ponds had lower SPC and DMSCC counts than other herds in the state with no access to ponds and those herds with natural ponds were higher in both categories. From these data it could be argued that people who built man-made ponds were better managers and thus had higher milk quality.

Chapter 3

Keeping Animals

Housing Buffalow

Housing for water buffaloes should give protection against thermal stress - particularly direct exposure to sun, heavy rains and cold weather. It must allow good ventilation. Housing may therefore be different in different areas of the world, due to differences in climate.

Below are some considerations and solutions when planning housing in hot and cold climates respectively. Common for all housing is that enough space should be allowed for each buffalo.

The outdoor yard should preferably be covered with grass or maybe concrete, in order to prevent it from becoming an unhygienic mud hole in rainy periods.

Hot climate

Buffaloes may appear to be misplaced in a hot and humid environment. They have a dark skin and few sweat glands and are more or less dependent on water for their cooling. This is not entirely true, buffaloes protected from direct sunlight do very well even during hot and humid days, partly because their ability to loose heat through the respiratory tract.

High milk production requires a high feed intake which leads to higher metabolic heat production. High yielding buffaloes thus have a disadvantage over lower yielding animals, and need more cooling facilities. The following points are guidelines to have in mind when giving advice on management.

- The feeding, watering and milking place should always give shade and protection from heavy rains, either by trees or by a roof.
- Cool water either from a clean river or served in an earthen pit, helps the animals to maintain temperature. Water trough should always be placed in the shade.
- A paddock with trees gives a very cheap and effective protection from sun. However, the trees may need to be protected from the buffaloes also.
- A shelter of a simple construction with only a roof. In hot humid climates it is better not to have walls. Walls may lead to inadequate ventilation and thereby favouring bacteria and mold growth, thus making the stable unhygienic. To protect the inside from sunshine (or heavy rain), curtains made from straw, textile or other suitable material, can be used.
- Providing the animals with a wallow. However, the wallow should be one with clean water and not far from the farm. Spending time walking in the sun to and from the wallowing costs more than it saves.
- Showering of the buffaloes with cool water for 3 minutes twice a day has proven to be an efficient way for them to get rid of excess heat.

Cold Climate

- A shelter should protect the animals from rain, snow and strong wind. It may be a simple construction with a roof and three walls. This system will allow the buffaloes to go outside to graze when the weather allows it. There should be a feeding area inside the shelter in case of several days with bad weather. A separate heated milking area is advisable in this case.
- A dry and clean bedding is important in cold weathers to maintain animal health.
- In case of extremely cold climate, (Caucasia and Balkan) with several months with a temperature below 0?C, a heated barn may be necessary.

Pens for Calves

Calves should be kept in individual pens for the first month. The pens should be easy to keep clean, with shelter from direct sunlight, rain, snow and draught. By keeping the calves individually it is easier to check that they eat and grow properly and to detect illnesses. Also, naval suckling is avoided and spread of diseases is more difficult.

The calves should have access to fresh and clean water at all times. Preferably, the buckets for milk and water should be outside the pen, in a steady holder within easy reach for the calf. Hereby, the calves can not splash it on the bedding. A humid bedding will facilitate growth of germs and parasites. The pen should contain a holder for hay and concentrate. These holders should be placed above the ground so that the calf cannot step or defecate in them.

Chicken coop

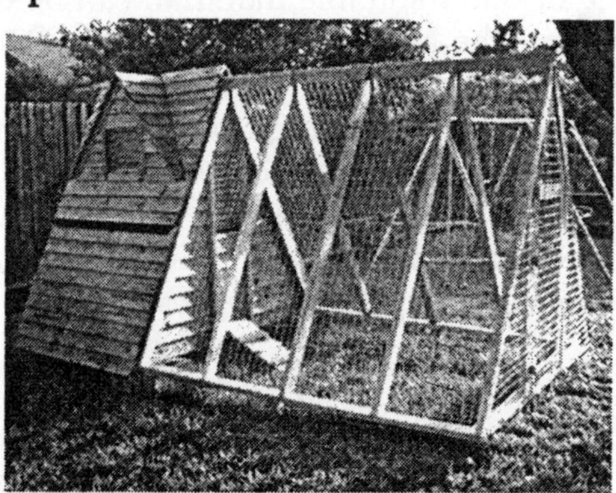

Fig. Chicken coop

A chicken coop is a building where chickens are kept on a farm or homestead. The inside of the chicken coop normally consists of several nesting boxes just large enough for the chickens to sit in while laying their eggs, as well as perches for the chickens to use while sleeping. Often the floor of the chicken coop is covered with a material, such as straw or wood chips, to contain the chicken waste, and to allow easier cleanup of the chicken coop. Sometimes the chicken coop contains feeding and watering devices for the chickens, but these may also be kept outside of the chicken coop. Most have some kind of ventilation to help air out any odors that may occur.

Since chickens are often prone to illness from drafts and poor weather, chicken coops are best designed to be warm at cold times, cool at hot times, and as draft free as possible. Many people, especially in rural areas, keep a small flock of chickens to provide themselves with eggs and meat. These small coops are often surrounded by a fence, usually made with wire fencing to allow the chickens an area to roam, peck, and hunt insects, to keep them contained. Contrary to popular use of the term, fencing known as "chicken wire" is often too weak to pose a barrier to predators and is therefore seldom used to confine the birds.

Free range

Free range poultry farming consists of poultry permitted to roam freely instead of being contained in any manner. The principle is to allow the animals as much freedom as possible, to live out their instinctual behaviours in a reasonably natural way, regardless of whether or not they are eventually killed for meat. In the UK, the Department for Environment, Food and Rural Affairs says that a free range chicken must have daytime access to open-air runs during at least half of their life. Unlike in the United States, this definition also applies to eggs. The European Union regulates marketing standards for egg farming which specifies a minimum condition for Free Range Eggs states that "hens have continuous daytime access to open-air runs, except in the case of temporary restrictions imposed by veterinary authorities".

NEST BOX

A nest box also called birdhouse is a man-made box provided for animals to nest in. Nest boxes are most frequently utilized for wild and domesticated birds, but certain species of mammal may also use them. Boxes are usually wooden, though some for birds are made from mixtures of wood and concrete, called *woodcrete*. Metal nest boxes are also marketed, but these are generally unsuitable for outdoor use, as they can overheat easily in sunshine. The majority are cuboid, and many have a sloping roof. Many have a hinged top to provide access for cleaning, bird ringing or, when used for domesticated species, to give the breeder access to the young. Boxes may either have an entrance hole or be open fronted. Some nest boxes can be highly decorated and complex. Designs mimicking human house design or other structures are common in some gardens.

The size of a nest box should be suited for the guest inside it. Quite large boxes are used for ducks and owls. Nest boxes for wild birds should be cleaned annually to remove old nests and kill parasites. The nest boxes of domestic birds and other animals should be removed and cleaned after the breeding season is over and no more young are expected. Budgerigars and other birds raised domestically will not usually mate unless a nest box is present. Bats houses are becoming popular sources of natural mosquito and insect control. A single bat can eat 500 to 1,000 mosquitoes a night as well as numerous garden pests.

Directions for making the open bottom bat houses for small and large colonies, as well as locations to purchase them are available on the internet. Bat houses are an ecologically friendly way of controlling mosquitoes as pesticides mostly kill the mosquito's predators rather than mosquitoes. Nest boxes are marketed not only for birds but also for bats, some other mammals and bees. Depending on the animal, these boxes are used for roosting, breeding, or both. Most small mammals will use a nest box for raising young if one is provided.

Kennel

A kennel is the name given to any structure or shelter for dogs. A *kennel* is a doghouse, run, or other small structure in which a dog is kept. American English often uses the word "doghouse" in this context; in British English the term "kennel" is preferred, but the phrase "in the doghouse" is understood but does not mean "in the kennel", rather it is a colloquial phrase meaning (of a person) "in trouble" or "being shunned".

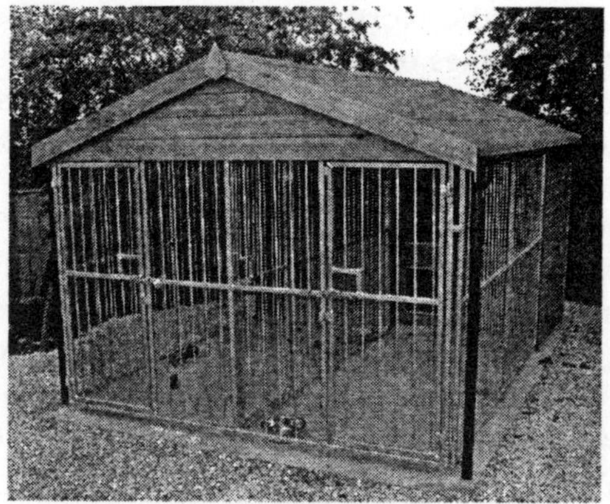

Fig. Kennel for Dog

Used in the plural, *the kennels*, the term means any building, collection of buildings or a property in which dogs are housed, maintained, and bred.

Stable

A stable is a building in which livestock, especially horses, are kept. It most commonly means a building that is divided into separate stalls for individual animals. There are many different types of stables in use today such as the American barn which is a large barn with a door each end and individual stalls inside or free standing stables with the classic top and bottom opening doors.

Historically, the headquarters of a unit of cavalry rather than just their horses' accommodation, would be called a stable.Used metaphorically from this origin, a stable is a collection of people (e.g. professional wrestlers) working under a single manager or animals kept by one owner.

Yarding

While often confused with free range farming, yarding is actually a separate method by which a hutch and fenced off area outside are combined when farming poultry. The distinction is that free-range poultry are either totally unfenced, or the fence is so distant that it has little influence on their freedom of movement. This is common technique used by small farms in the Northeastern portion of the US. Daily releases out of hutches or coops allows for instinctuial nature for the chickens with protections from predators. The hens usually lay eggs either on the ground of the coop or in baskets if provided by the farmer.

This technique can be complicated if used with roosters though, mostly because of difficulty getting them into the coop and to clean the coop while it is inside. This territorial nature is apparent while outside in which they have a brood of hens and sometimes even informal land claims. This can endanger people unaware of the existence of the territories who are attacked by the larger birds.

Housing goats

Housing for dairy goats does not have to be elaborate, but it must satisfy the health and comfort of the animals. There are five requirements of good housing for goats:

- The building should be adequately ventilated but not drafty;
- The walls and ceiling should be free from condensation;
- The bedded area should be relatively dry and clean;
- The hay, grain and water receptacles must be well built and located so that feed is not wasted or contaminated; and
- The facilities should provide easy access to the animals and require a minimum amount of labour.

The comfort zone for dairy goats is between 55 and 70 degrees Fahrenheit. Non-sweating animals are much less sensitive to declining temperatures than to rising temperatures. Milk production, feed consumption and comfort are not affected by temperatures between 0 and 55 degrees Fahrenheit, but temperatures over 80 degrees Fahrenheit seriously reduce feed intake and milk output. Therefore, the object is not how to keep the goats warm in winter, but how to keep them cool in summer.

The movement of air, either by mechanical or natural means, to remove heat, moisture and odors is a necessary part of a housing plan. Most pneumonia problems with dairy goats can be traced to inadequate ventilation. Wet walls and ceilings are the result of improper ventilation, poor insulation or a combination of the two. The rate of air movement is influenced by the amount of animal heat produced and the temperature you wish to maintain in the building. Additional heat and insulation may be required to keep the stable air fresh and to prevent water pipes from freezing in the winter. An air inlet system also must be provided for good air distribution. Ventilation entails more than installing a fan to move some air.

Proper ventilation during the summer may require moving 150 to 200 cubic feet of air per minute per animal. Winter weather may reduce the amount of air to be exhausted to as little as 20 cubic feet per goat. Contact your local MU Extension specialist for assistance in planning the right ventilation system.

With proper ventilation, you are protecting the animals, the building and the quality of milk produced. Windows are essential in a closed barn. They permit sunlight for warmth and drying and provide a source of vitamin D for the animals. Well-lighted barns usually are kept cleaner. In summer, open windows are important for air movement.

Housing for Young Stock and the Milking Herd

There are two housing systems often used for goats:

- Loose housing, where the animals run loose in a pen or shed
- Stall barns, where each animal is confined in a small box stall or tie stall

Loose housing is an old system with many desirable features. With plenty of bedding, the manure pack for a goat herd can be kept fairly clean and dry. Heat produced within the pack makes a warm bed. There is ample exercise area and an opportunity for the goats to move around.

This type of housing, however, presents a few problems. A built-up manure pack, even though dry on the surface, releases a lot of moisture into the barn air. In addition, hay racks should be located off the bedded area to reduce parasite infestations. Watering devices should be placed in an area where spilled water will not mess up the bedded pack. Many goat owners use a shed or barn that is open on the south or southeast side, thus eliminating the need for mechanical ventilation.

These are cold housing facilities that do not require additional heat or insulation and use normal air movement for ventilation. Goats move freely in or out of the housing area and into the paddock or feeding area. Hay feeders, watering devices, mineral feeders and grain bunks are located on concrete pads some distance from the built-up manure pack.

Housing for the kids and other young stock may be included in the plan for the milking herd. However, young goats must be kept separate from the milking herd. Frequently, the kids are kept in 4-foot-square box stalls with at least one side slatted to permit air movement. Do not make a box stall from plywood with all four walls solid; air movement will not reach the kids.

Usually a gated front contains enough openings to allow air drainage. Provide a heat lamp for newborn kids and for kids that are ill. Older kids may be kept in a corner of the stable area inside a pen made from movable hurdles. Buck housing must be separate and downwind from the milking herd. It does not have to be elaborate and often is no more than a 5- or 6-foot shed with an open side facing the south to give the bucks free access to an exercise lot.

The milking area is part of the housing plan, but it should be separated from the stable area. It should have a concrete floor to make cleaning easier, and the milking platform should be 15 to 18 inches higher than the floor to permit easier milking. The platform should allow 18 inches in width and 3-1/2 feet in length for each animal to be tied. The manger should be 6 inches deep and 1 foot wide. If several goats are to be fastened and milked at once, a lever that will open and close the stanchion head locks is helpful.

Some goat owners who keep their milking herds in stall barns milk their animals on a milking stand located in one corner of the stable. Dusty air and flies in the stable, however, may require you to place the milking stand in a separate screened-in facility to guarantee clean milk. A 5-by-8-foot room with a concrete floor and drain is adequate for milking a small herd, but be sure there is plenty of light either from natural sources or electric bulbs.

If the milk is sold to the public or to a processor, there will be state inspection of the operation just as is required for production of Grade A milk from cows. Check with your local health authorities and the state inspector before starting construction.If the milk is to be used by the family, the degree of sanitation and cleanliness maintained and the size and type of building constructed can be based on the owner's good sense, pride, conscience and finances. Equip the milk house with a double sink for washing utensils, a hot water heater, refrigeration, a small table or work space, and a rack for drying and storing utensils. At least 50 percent of the milk house should be open floor space with ample room for equipment.

Regardless of the herd size, refrigeration must be available to quickly cool the milk. A household refrigerator may be used, but cold water is more efficient in cooling milk than cold air. The refrigerator or cooler should be large enough to hold a pan of water. The pan should hold enough water to match the amount of milk in the milk bucket. If the herd is big enough and milk production is 5, 10 or more gallons per day, it will be necessary to purchase a water-immersion cooler or a bulk tank for cooling purposes.

Cooling is critical to milk flavor and quality. All milk contains bacteria, some of which comes from the air and the utensils. If milk remains warm for a short period, the bacteria begin to multiply and the quality of milk deteriorates. Therefore, cool milk immediately after milking to a temperature under 40 degrees Fahrenheit and hold it at that temperature until processed and/or consumed. Plans for building a milking barn and milking stand and for construction of the milk house area are available from your local MU Extension dairy specialist.

Fences serve two purposes that make them an important

part of a housing plan — they keep goats in and dogs out. They also keep foraging goats away from your trees and shrubs as well as your neighbour's flower patch. Set 7-foot posts, either wooden or steel, on 12-foot centres.

Then use either a 4-foot-high woven wire fence topped with an electric wire 12 inches above the woven wire or use a completely electric fence. If you use a completely electric fence, place the first wire 12 inches from the ground, then four more wires on 6-inch spacings to a total height of 36 inches. Use insulators on the post to attach the wires. The electric fence works well when weeds, grass and brush are not allowed to touch the wires and short it out or when the ground isn't bone dry during periods of drought. Your local farm supply store can recommend the proper equipment.

In summary, keep the plans as simple and economical as possible. Consider the health of your animals as well as the conveniences a housing facility might offer. Contact your local MU Extension specialist for additional ideas on housing facilities for your dairy goat enterprise.

BEEKEEPING

Fixed Frame Hives

There are considerable regional variations in the type of hive in which bees are kept. A hive is a set of rectangular wooden boxes filled with moveable wood or plastic frames, each of which holds a sheet of wax or plastic foundation. The bees build cells upon the sheets of foundation to create complete honeycombs. Foundation comes in two cell-sizes: worker foundation - which enables the bees to create small, hexagonal worker cells and 'drone foundation' which allows the bees to build much larger cells - drone cells, for the production of male bees.

The bottom box, or brood chamber, contains the queen and most of the bees; the upper boxes, or supers, contain just honey. Only the young nurse bees can produce wax flakes which they secrete from between their abdominal plates; they build honeycomb using the artificial wax foundation as a starting point, after which they may raise brood or deposit honey and pollen in the cells of the comb. These frames can be freely manipulated and honey supers with frames full of honey can be taken and extracted for their honey crop.

MODERN BEEKEEPING

Movable Frame Hives

In the USA, the Langstroth hive is commonly used. The Langstroth was the first successful top-opened hive with movable frames, and other designs of hive have been based on it. Langstroth hive was however a descendant of Jan Dzierzon's Polish hive designs. In the United Kingdom, the most common type of hive is the British National Hive, but it is not unusual to see some other sorts of hive.

Straw skeps, bee gums, and unframed box hives are now unlawful in most US states, as the comb and brood cannot be inspected for diseases. However, straw skeps are still used for collecting swarms by hobbyists in the UK, before moving them into standard hives.

Top Bar Hives

A few hobby beekeepers are adopting various top bar hives of the type commonly found in Africa. These have no frames and the honey filled comb is not returned to the hive after extraction, as it is in the Langstroth hive. Because of this, the production of honey in a top bar hive is only about 20 per cent that of a Langstroth hive, but the initial costs and equipment requirements are far lower.

Top-bar hives also offer some advantages in interacting with the bees and the amount of weight that must be lifted is greatly reduced. Top Bar Hives are being widely used in developing countries in Africa and Asia as a result of 'Bees For Development' programme.

Protective Clothing

Beekeepers often wear protective clothing to protect themselves from stings. While knowledge of the bees is the first line of defence, most beekeepers also wear some protective clothing. Novice beekeepers usually wear gloves and a hooded suit or hat and veil. Experienced beekeepers sometimes elect not to use gloves because they inhibit delicate manipulations. The face and neck are the most important areas to protect, so most beekeepers will at least wear a veil.

Defensive bees are attracted to the breath, and a sting on the face can lead to much more pain and swelling than a sting elsewhere, while a sting on a bare hand can usually be quickly removed by fingernail scrape to reduce the amount of venom injected.

The protective clothing is generally light coloured and of a smooth material. This provides the maximum differentiation from the colony's natural predators (bears, skunks, etc.) which tend to be dark-coloured and furry.

AQUACULTURE

Aquaculture is the cultivation of aquatic organisms. Unlike fishing, aquaculture, also known as aquafarming, implies the cultivation of aquatic populations under controlled conditions. Mariculture refers to aquaculture practiced in marine environments. Particular kinds of aquaculture include algaculture (the production of kelp/seaweed and other algae); fish farming; shrimp farming, shellfish farming, and the growing of cultured pearls.

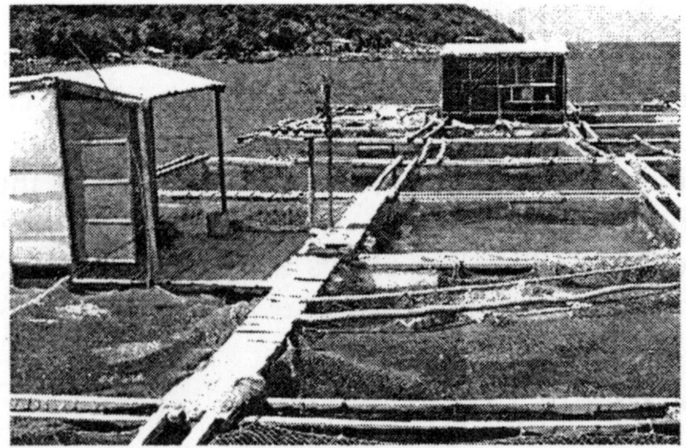

Fig. Aquaculture

Aquaculture has been used in China since circa 2500 BC.

When the waters lowered after river floods, some fishes, namely carp, were held in artificial lakes. Their brood were later fed using nymphs and silkworm feces, while the fish themselves were eaten as a source of protein. By a fortunate genetic mutation, this early domestication of carp lead to the development of goldfish in the Tang Dynasty.

The Hawaiian people practiced aquaculture by constructing fish ponds. A remarkable example from ancient Hawaii is the construction of a fish pond, dating from at least 1,000 years ago, at Alekoko. According to legend, it was constructed by the mythical Menehune. The Japanese practiced cultivation of seaweed by providing bamboo poles and, later, nets and oyster shells to serve as anchoring surfaces for spores. The Romans often bred fish in ponds.

The practice of aquaculture gained prevalence in Europe during the Middle Ages, since fish were scarce and thus expensive. However, improvements in transportation during the 19th century made fish easily available and inexpensive, even in inland areas, causing a decline in the practice.

The first North American fish hatchery was constructed on Dildo Island, Newfoundland Canada in 1889, it was the largest and most advanced in the world. Americans were rarely involved in aquaculture until the late 20th century, but California residents harvested wild kelp and made legal efforts to manage the supply starting circa 1900, later even producing it as a wartime resource.

In contrast to agriculture, the rise of aquaculture is a contemporary phenomenon. According to professor Carlos M. Duarte About 430 (97 per cent) of the aquatic species presently in culture have been domesticated since the start of the 20th century, and an estimated 106 aquatic species have been domesticated over the past decade. The domestication of an aquatic species typically involves about a decade of scientific research.

Current success in the domestication of aquatic species results from the 20th century rise of knowledge on the basic biology of aquatic species and the lessons learned from past success and failure. The stagnation in the world's fisheries and overexploitation of 20 to 30 per cent of marine fish species have provided additional impetus to domesticate marine species, just as overexploitation of land animals provided the impetus for the early domestication of land species

In the 1960s, the price of fish began to climb, as wild fish capture rates peaked and the human population continued to rise. Today, commercial aquaculture exists on an unprecedented, huge scale. In the 1980s, open-netcage salmon farming also expanded; this particular type of aquaculture technology remains a minor part of the production of farmed finfish worldwide, but possible negative impacts on wild stocks, which have come into question since the late 1990s, have caused it to become a major cause of controversy.

TYPES OF AQUACULTURE

Algaculture

Algaculture is a form of aquaculture involving the farming of species of algae. The majority of algae that are intentionally cultivated fall into the category of microalgae, also referred to as phytoplankton, microphytes, or planktonic algae. Macroalgae, commonly know as seaweed, also have many commercial and industrial uses, but due to their size and the specific requirements of the environment in which they need to grow, they do not lend themselves as readily to cultivation on a large scale as microalgae and are most often harvested wild from the ocean.

Fish Farming

Fish farming is the principal form of aquaculture, while other methods may fall under mariculture. It involves raising fish commercially in tanks or enclosures, usually for food. A facility that releases juvenile fish into the wild for recreational fishing or to supplement a species' natural numbers is generally referred to as a fish hatchery.

Fish species raised by fish farms include salmon, catfish, tilapia, cod, carp, trout and others. Increasing demands on wild fisheries by commercial fishing operations have caused widespread overfishing. Fish farming offers an alternative solution to the increasing market demand for fish and fish protein.

Freshwater Prawn Farming

A freshwater prawn farm is an aquaculture business designed to raise and produce freshwater prawn or shrimp for human consumption. Freshwater prawn farming shares many characteristics with, and many of the same problems as, marine shrimp farming.

Unique problems are introduced by the developmental life cycle of the main species. The global annual production of freshwater prawns (excluding crayfish and crabs) in 2003 was about 280,000 tons, of which China produced some 180,000 tons, followed by India and Thailand with some 35,000 tons each. Additionally, China produced about 370,000 tons of Chinese river crab (*Eriocheir sinensis*).

Integrated Multi-trophic Aquaculture

Integrated Multi-Trophic Aquaculture (IMTA) is a practice in which the by-products (wastes) from one species are recycled to become inputs (fertilizers, food) for another. Fed aquaculture is combined with inorganic extractive (e.g. seaweed) and organic extractive (e.g. shellfish) aquaculture to create balanced systems for environmental sustainability (biomitigation), economic stability (product diversification and risk reduction) and social acceptability (better management practices).

"Multi-Trophic" refers to the incorporation of species from different trophic or nutritional levels in the same system. This is one potential distinction from the age-old practice of aquatic polyculture, which could simply be the co-culture of different fish species from the same trophic level. In this case, these organisms may all share the same biological and chemical processes, with few synergistic benefits, which could potentially lead to significant shifts in the ecosystem.

Some traditional polyculture systems may, in fact, incorporate a greater diversity of species, occupying several niches, as extensive cultures (low intensity, low management) within the same pond. The "Integrated" in IMTA refers to the more intensive cultivation of the different species in proximity of each other, connected by nutrient and energy transfer through water, but not necessarily right at the same location.

Ideally, the biological and chemical processes in an IMTA system should balance. This is achieved through the appropriate selection and proportions of different species providing different ecosystem functions.

The co-cultured species should be more than just biofilters; they should also be harvestable crops of commercial value. A working IMTA system should result in greater production for the overall system, based on mutual benefits to the co-cultured species and improved ecosystem health, even if the individual production of some of the species is lower compared to what could be reached in monoculture practices over a short term period.

Sometimes the more general term "Integrated Aquaculture" is used to describe the integration of monocultures through water transfer between organisms. For all intents and purposes however, the terms "IMTA" and "integrated aquaculture" differ primarily in their degree of descriptiveness. These terms are sometimes interchanged. Aquaponics, fractionated aquaculture, IAAS (integrated agriculture-aquaculture systems), IPUAS (integrated peri-urban-aquaculture systems), and IFAS (integrated fisheries-aquaculture systems) may also be considered variations of the IMTA concept.

Mariculture

Mariculture is a specialized branch of aquaculture involving the cultivation of marine organisms for food and other products in the open ocean, an enclosed section of the ocean, or in tanks, ponds or raceways which are filled with seawater. An example of the latter is the farming of marine fish, prawns, or oysters in saltwater ponds. Non-food products produced by mariculture include: fish meal, nutrient agar, jewelries (e.g. cultured pearls), and cosmetics.

Shrimp Farming

A shrimp farm is an aquaculture business for the cultivation of marine shrimp for human consumption. Commercial shrimp farming began in the 1970s, and production grew steeply, particularly to match the market demands of the U.S., Japan and Western Europe. The total global production of farmed shrimp reached more than 1.6 million tonnes in 2003, representing a value of nearly 9,000 million U.S. dollars. About 75 per cent of farmed shrimp is produced in Asia, in particular in China and Thailand. The other 25 per cent is produced mainly in Latin America, where Brazil is the largest producer. The largest exporting nation is Thailand.

Shrimp farming has changed from traditional, small-scale businesses in Southeast Asia into a global industry. Technological advances have led to growing shrimp at ever higher densities, and broodstock is shipped world-wide. Virtually all farmed shrimp are penaeids (i.e., shrimp of the family *Penaeidae*), and just two species of shrimp—the *Penaeus vannamei* (Pacific white shrimp) and the *Penaeus monodon* (giant tiger prawn)—account for roughly 80 per cent of all farmed shrimp.

These industrial monocultures are very susceptible to diseases, which have caused several regional wipe-outs of farm shrimp populations. Increasing ecological problems, repeated disease outbreaks, and pressure and criticism from both NGOs and consumer countries led to changes in the industry in the late 1990s and generally stronger regulation by governments. In 1999, a programme aimed at developing and promoting more sustainable farming practices was initiated, including governmental bodies, industry representatives, and environmental organizations.

Chapter 4

Animal Breeding

The science of Animal breeding is defined as the application of the principles of Genetics and biometry to improve the efficiency of production in farm animals. These principles were applied to change animal populations thousands of years before the sciences of genetics and biometry were formally established. The practice of animal breeding dates back to the Neolithic period, when people attempted to domesticate wild species such as reindeer, goats, hogs and dogs.

Domestication was performed through controlled mating and reproduction of captive animals which were selected and mated based on their behaviour and temperament. Judging from cave paintings that have survived, selection was also applied to some qualitative traits such as coat colour and the absence or presence of horns.

Without written records, there is no certain knowledge of the evolution of animal breeding practices, but written documents dating back more than 4000 years indicate that humans appreciated the significance of family resemblance in mating systems, recognized the dangers of intense inbreeding, and used castration to prevent the reproduction of undesirable males. Progress in the performance of domesticated animals through these selection practices was very slow; improvements were mainly due to animals adapting better to their environments.

Robert Bakewell, an English animal breeder of the 18th century, is considered the founder of systematized animal breeding. He was the first to emphasize the importance of accurate breeding records, introduced the concept of progeny testing to evaluate the genetic potentials of young sires, and applied inbreeding to stabilize desired qualitative traits. He also promoted concepts such as "like begets like," "prepotency is associated with inbreeding" and "breed the best to the best." Bakewell and his contemporaries in Europe pioneered the development of diverse breeds of Beef cattle, Dairy cattle, Sheep. Colour, conformation, geographical origin and some production characteristics were the main factors that differentiated these breeds. Wide geographical redistribution of animal populations was also an important factor in the formation of new breeds, as invading armies, migrating people and traders transported livestock to new lands.

Animal breeding as a modern science belongs to the 20th century. Although numerous geneticists and biometricians have made significant contributions to the development of this science, J.L. Lush of Iowa State University is considered the father of the modern science of animal breeding. Lush and his students developed major scientific procedures applicable to the genetic improvement of farm animals.

SELECTIVE BREEDING

Selective breeding in domesticated animals is the process of a breeder developing a cultivated breed over time, and selecting qualities within individuals of the breed that will be best to pass on to the next generation. Breeding techniques such as inbreeding, linebreeding and outcrossing are utilized by breeders in the maintenance and improvement of their chosen breeds.

Breeding Stock

"Breeding stock" is a term used to describe a group of animals used for purpose of planned breeding. When an individual is looking to breed animals, he or she is looking for certain valuable traits in purebred stock for a certain purpose, or may intend to use some type of crossbreeding to produce a new type of stock with different, and presumably superior abilities in a given area of endeavor.

To breed chickens, a typical breeder intends to receive eggs, meat, and new, young birds for further reproduction. Thus the breeder has to study different breeds and types of chickens and analyse what can be expected from a certain set of characteristics before he or she starts breeding them. Accordingly, when purchasing initial breeding stock, the breeder seeks a group of birds that will most closely fit the purpose intended.

Purebred Breeding

The idea of *breed purity* may strike an unpleasant chord with some individuals because it is reminiscent of nineteenth-century eugenics notions of a "superior strain" in humans, supposedly exemplified by members of an aristocratic social class or of certain races. The application of theories of eugenics had far-reaching consequences for human beings, particularly in cases such as The Holocaust.

However, the idea of a superior strain in animals, such as that incorporated in the breeding of Thoroughbred race horses, was less controversial. By "breeding the best to the best," employing a certain degree of careful inbreeding, considerable culling, and selection for "superior" qualities, one could develop a bloodline or "breed" superior in certain respects to the original base stock or landrace which had been produced primarily by natural selection.

This process forms the basis for a "true-breeding" line of animals, which today is generally called a "purebred" line. Once created, a purified line is "closed" and preserved from dilution and possible "debasement" by unrelated stock.

However, this theory is not without some negative consequences. When the ideal of purified lineage or purely aesthetic type is seen as an end in itself, without consideration of usefulness or vigour, a breed can suffer over time. Also, if a breed registry is closed with too small a gene pool, over time, degradation due to inbreeding depression may occur. For many purebred breeders, the need for a periodic outcross is recognized and incorporated into an overall plan.

The observable phenomenon of hybrid vigour stands in

contrast to the notion of breed purity. However, on the other hand, indiscriminate breeding of crossbred or hybrid animals may also result in degradation of quality, particularly when animals are mass-produced without concern for overall health or longevity.

Backyard Breeding

The term backyard breeder is a general term, sometimes considered derisive, used to describe people who are "home breeders", and breed only a few animals for personal use or occasional sale. However, while some backyard breeders pay strict attention to quality, the term usually describes those who allow animals, particularly dogs or horses, to procreate regardless of physical, genetic, and/or emotional health.

It is also used to describe unreputable commercial breeders. In the process of careless breeding, many backyard breeders produce genetically weak animals that can be predisposed to genetic disorders or debilitating physical deformities, particularly those that result from inbreeding.

In dog breeding, these individuals focus on only a limited aspect of the dog, while ignoring the original function and temperament of the breed. When such breeding is carried out on a large scale, the venue is called a *puppy mill* or *puppy farm.* Backyard breeding is popularly blamed for the proliferation of aggressive dogs for the sports of dog baiting and dog fighting. Dog fanciers generally believe that such ill-bred dogs are the reason for the bad public reputation of certain dog breeds, and the increasingly frequent enactment of breed-specific legislation.

Because of the time and expense of feeding and caring for horses, which produce one foal per year, there are fewer horse breeders who produce animals *en masse,* though some individuals do engage in animal hoarding and breed far more animals than they can support. In the horse world, over breeding of grade animals that cannot be sold except for very low prices raises concerns that such animals will be slaughtered for horsemeat.

Some, though not all, colour breeders make errors similar

to puppy mill breeders by focusing on only one characteristic to the detriment of health, soundness, and quality conformation. In addition, industrial breeders, such as those who produce *pregnant mare urine* for the manufacture of premarin, allow many mares to be bred indiscriminately, simply so that they are able to produce the urine laced with reproductive hormones that forms the base for the drug. Their foals are generally considered an unwanted byproduct, particularly males (colts), and sold off, frequently to the slaughter market.

IN-BREEDING AND OTHER BREEDING METHODS

One of the most hotly talked about topics with regard to pure-bred dogs is the use of in-breeding. This is a term that is often misused and is extremely misunderstood.

Part of the misunderstandings comes from differences in the way the terms are used within the scientific/medical field, and how it is commonly used by breeders. These are the most commonly accepted definitions used by serious dog breeders and will be the definitions used within this article.

In-breeding: This is the breeding of closely related animals. Brother-Sister, Parent-Offspring.

Line-breeding: This is the breeding of animals that share common ancestors but are not closely related. The dogs may share a common great-grandparent.

Out-cross: This is generally considered the breeding of animals with no common ancestors within the first 4 or 5 generations.

Common Misconceptions

In-breeding causes genetic diseases: Breeding closely related animals increases the possibility that any bad genes in a line will show up. It does not 'cause' genetic disease.

Out-crossed dogs are healthier: This is only partly true. There is a known phenomenon called Hybrid Vigour. Two animals of unrelated strains breed and the offspring is often bigger and grows faster than it's purebred cousins. This method is often used by farmers in order to get their animals to market sooner.

But one of the biggest misconceptions of hybrid vigour is that it applies to all animals of mixed heritage. Hybrid Vigour only applies to the animals that are the direct offspring of the crossing of the unrelated strains. In other words if you continue to breed animals of different strains there generally will not be any additional increase in hybrid vigour.

If the unrelated strains share common genes for genetic disorders, hybrid vigour will not over ride the risk of the disorder showing up. Out-crossing can also cause problems if widely divergent physical types are mixed due to differences in growth rates and bone and muscle sizes.

BENEFITS OF EACH TYPE OF BREEDING

By definition, purebred dogs have a smaller gene pool to draw on than mixed breed dogs. That smaller gene pool gives the breed its individual characteristics, such as physical appearance and temperament. It is what makes a poodle a Poodle and a Golden Retriever a Golden Retriever. But there is considerable controversy with regard to whether the gene pools of the modern pure-bred have become too small.

Inbreeding

In-breeding is more likely to help "set" or "fix" a particular trait within a breed or a line by narrowing the gene pool to favour those traits. So if a breeder is looking to set a particular desirable feature of their line then in-breeding and choosing the offspring most strongly possessing that trait can be beneficial.

In the first pedigree Sydney is the maternal son of Annie, thus doubling on Annie's genes. Or another way to look at it is Annie is both Sydney's mother and Grand-mother. In the second example we have a full brother/sister in-breeding so we are doubling up on the genes from both Kiley and Annie.

In-breeding can also help identify those bad genes that exist within a line. Dogs possessing the bad genes can be eliminated from a breeding programme and carriers also identified.

Intermittent in-breeding within a line or breed is not

damaging to the long term health of the animals. However, in-breeding over successive generations can lead to reduced fitness and fertility problems among the offspring, resulting in phenomena known as In-breeding Depression. It can take many generations to show up depending on the traits involved.

To use this method responsibly a breeder would not want to in-breed on animals with known genetic disorders, temperaments not in keeping with its given breed, or known serious structural faults, or to in-breed frequently even on healthy-superior specimens.

Line-Breeding

Line-breeding is another way to help "set" or "fix" desirable traits. With line-breeding we breed animals that are related, but we are also routinely introducing genes from other lines into the genetic mix. It takes longer to fix the desirable traits this way, but doing so lowers the risk of those problems associated with repeated in-breeding.

Loose line-breeding over successive generations will result in more variations of physical appearance than would in-breeding or tight line-breeding, but will keep the physical look and structure within the same general size and shape, it also carries fewer long term risks.

According to geneticists: Line-breeding can be carried on for many many generations without deleterious effects on the line or breed as long as the individuals involved have few hidden genetic disorders.

Out-Crossing

Out-crossing in terms of pure-bred dogs is the breeding of unrelated dogs. On a pedigree no names will be repeated within the first 5 generations.

This type of breeding has both advantages and disadvantages. Which as it turns out are flip sides of the same argument. The greatest genetic diversity are maintained by out -ccrossing, but this also leads to the least consistency in terms of physical appearance and other traits.

Out-crossing does not guarantee that the animals won't develop genetic disorders, but it does tend to reduce the numbers of affected offspring. Best chance of getting an animal that is less prone to developing a genetic disorder comes more from finding a conscientious breeder that screens their animals for hereditary disorders and breeds for the betterment of the breed.

All three methods of breeding have their place in a long term, well thought out breeding programme. Talk to the breeder, ask questions as to what their goal is in doing a particular breeding. Ask about the risks and what problems are known to that line. And all lines have some because the perfect dog and the perfect lines are still goals of the future for all breeders.

COW BREEDING

Different Breeds for Different Needs

Dairy cattle are breeds that have been developed to produce milk whereas beef cattle are bred and selected primarily for the production of meat. Dual-purpose breeds do exist and they have been selected for both meat and milk production. In the last 20 years the genetic make up of the UK dairy herd has changed and is still changing. Cows are larger, earlier maturing, are producing far more milk and are more efficient at converting feed into milk.

As it is the birth of the calf that causes milk production, it is critical for the farmer that the cow becomes pregnant again during lactation and produces the next calf one year after the previous one. The average length of productive life of a dairy cow is between four and five lactations, although this varies from one or two to over ten.

Since the fifties artificial insemination (AI) has increasingly replaced natural service. Embryo transplants (ET) are also being developed. A surrogate mother may have difficulty delivering, since the foreign calf is often larger than nature intended. When this happens, a rope or chain is attached to the calf's forelegs, and, with a winch-like device the newborn calf is pulled from the womb. Unnecessary suffering for both cow and calf.

Regular Calving

A high annual milk production per cow is dependent on regular calving at about 12- month intervals. Poor reproductive efficiency leads to longer calving indices and a reduction in milk sales per cow per annum. It also leads to an increase in the number of cows culled for failing to conceive. On average, in the UK, only about 85 cows calve per annum for every 100 cows available for breeding. Over thirty-five per cent of all cows culled are disposed of because of reproductive disorders.

Obtaining Semen

Photographer Henry Heap visited the Milk Marketing Board stud bull operation in Mid Wales. He provided Turning Point magazine with a complete set of photographs and commentary of his visit. "A large, handsome, tan bull stood stock still, tethered by the ring tethered through his nose to what looked like a giant circular clothes line or some grotesque merry-go-round. He was kept so motionless by a rubber hood that covered his eyes, which had a similar effect to that of hooding a falcon.

A worker commented that the bull would stay still all day if they left the blindfold on. However, this bull was not the source of the semen, but instead what is known as a 'teaser'. The stud bulls are led out by the nose one at a time to mount the motionless hooded bull. After they have mounted the teaser their penis is diverted into a leather vagina which is used to collect the semen. As soon as the process is complete, another bull is led out. The hood keeps the teaser bull stationery for each successive beast to mount. These stud bulls never even see females.

During embryo transfer an embryo can be flushed from the uterus of a genetically superior cow and implanted in a receiver cow of so-called 'poorer quality' for foetal development. Embryos are also taken from dead cows at the slaughterhouse. Hormone treatment is used to induce multiple ovulations and the cow is then inseminated. A few days later several embryos can be flushed from her. For both embryo collection and implanting the cow receives a local anaesthetic injection in the tail. Embryos of the desired breed can then be used. ET maximises the number of offspring from selected breeding females and maximises profit.

Do-it-yourself embryo transfer is now taking place in the UK. Courses are run to train in direct embryo transfer techniques using the quick-thaw method for frozen embryos. Although vets are not required to be present at the time of transfer, they must check each animal is suitable for implantation. Farmers genetically improve the herd by using techniques such as MOET (multiple ovulation embryo transfer) which involves inducing a genetically 'superior' cow to produce up to 20 embryos rather than one.

For ease of management, farmers prefer cows to calf at the same time. They, therefore, need to detect when cows come into oestrous. The oestrous detection rate (ODR) is the number of cows observed in oestrus during a 3 week period, in relation to the number of cows expected to be observed. The average ODR on farms is about 60 per cent. One alternative is to synchronise the oestrous period of several animals by injections of prostaglandin or administration of progesterone as an impregnated intraveginal coil implanted for 9-12 days.

ARTIFICIAL INSEMINATION

Artificial insemination (AI) now accounts for around 75 per cent of British cattle births. The cow is tied up and one hand of the inseminator manipulates the cervix through the rectum wall whilst the other discharges semen into the vagina and cervix using an inseminating gun.

A regional manager with AI firm Genus the problems associated with the procedure. "Placing a quarter of a cc of diluted semen into an area as small as a penny coin, when the target area is inside 500kg of unco-operative cow, requires a high degree of expertise. The more the cow is able to move about, the harder it becomes to hit the target. Poor handling facilities cause stress, the cow, the inseminator and both our bank balances." There are many invasive procedures carried out on farm animals that the general public rarely witness. One of many includes making sure the cow is in calf. This is carried out using an ultrasound device much like a small TV set with a long thick wire attachment. A vet will insert their hand and arms length into the vagina of the cow.

The animal is held in a holding device to keep her still. The screen shows the small calf in the middle of a dark shaped uterus. Herds usually calve at the same time (due to human intervention) so all the cows on the farm will usually be checked at the same time.

Jersey Cattle

A small, honey-brown breed of dairy cattle, the Jersey is renowned for the high butterfat content of its milk, as well as a genial disposition.

The Jersey cow is quite small, ranging from only 800 to 1200 pounds (360 to 540 kg). The main factor contributing to the popularity of the breed has been their greater economy of production, due to:

- The ability to carry a larger number of effective milking cows per unit area due to lower body weight, hence lower maintenance requirements
- High butterfat conditions, and to thrive on locally produced food.

Bulls are also small, ranging from 1200 to 1800 pounds (540 to 820 kg), and are notoriously very aggressive. Castrated males can be trained into fine oxen which, due to their small size and gentle nature make them popular with young teamsters. Jersey oxen are not as strong as larger breeds however and are generally out of favour among competitive teamsters. Due to the small size, curious docile character and attractive features of the Jersey cow, small herds were imported into England by aristocratic landowners as props for aesthetic landscapes.

As its name implies, the Jersey was bred on the British Channel Island of Jersey. It apparently descended from cattle stock brought over from the nearby Norman mainland, and was first recorded as a separate breed around 1700. Frank Falle has speculated (on the basis of DNA evidence) that the oldest settlers in Jersey were Danish vikings who had been to Nantes with Hatain, where it is recorded that tribute was given by the King of France to Hatain of 500 cattle to leave that area, whereupon they settled in the Normandy area.

The marked resemblance between Jersey cattle and the Nantaise cow would seem to bear this out. While the breed is isolated from outside influence today, this was not always the case. Before 1789 cows would be given as dowry for inter-island marriages between Jersey and Guernsey. This was, however, not widespread.

Since 1789, imports of foreign cattle into Jersey have been forbidden by law to maintain the purity of the breed, although exports of cattle and semen have been an important economic resource for the island. The restriction on the import of cattle was initially introduced in 1789 to prevent a collapse in the export price. The United Kingdom levied no import duty on cattle imported from Jersey.

Cattle were being shipped from France to Jersey and then being shipped onward to England to circumvent the tariff on French cattle. The increase in the supply of cattle, sometimes of inferior quality, was bringing the price down and damaging the reputation of Jersey cattle. The import ban stabilised the price and enabled a more scientifically controlled programme of breeding to be undertaken.

Sheep Breeds

The domestic sheep is a multi-purpose animal, and the more than 200 breeds now in existence were created to serve these diverse purposes. Some sources give a count of a thousand or more breeds, but concrete documentation has not been produced for such a number. Almost all sheep are classified as being best suited to furnishing a certain product: wool, meat, milk, hides or a combination thereof (i.e. dual-purpose breeds).

Other features that are important when classifying sheep include face colour (generally white or black), the length of the tail, the presence or lack of horns, and the topography for which the breed has been developed. This last point is especially stressed in the United Kingdom, where breeds are described as either upland (hill or mountain) or lowland breeds. A sheep may also be of a fat-tailed breed, which is a type of dual-purpose sheep common in Africa and Asia with larger deposits of fat within its tail, or the meat from such a breed.

Ovine breeds are also grouped based on how well they are suited to producing a certain type of breeding stock. Generally, sheep are thought to be either "ewe breeds" or "ram breeds". Ewe breeds are those that are hardy, and have good reproductive and mothering capabilities—they are for replacing breeding ewes in standing flocks.

Ram breeds are selected for rate of weight gain and carcass quality, and are mated with ewe breeds to produce meat lambs. Many breeds, especially rare or primitive ones, fall into neither category strictly. Lowland and upland breeds are also crossed in this fashion, with the hardy hill ewes crossed with larger, fast-growing lowland rams to produce a type of ewe called a mule, which can then be crossed with meat-type rams to produce prime market lambs.

Sheep breeds are categorized by the type of wool they exhibit, irrespective of whether they are favoured for meat or wool production. Fine wool breeds are those that have wool of great crimp and density, and are consequently preferred by the textile industry. Most of these breeds were derived from Merino sheep, and Merinos continue to dominate the world sheep industry. The record for the most valuable sheep ever belongs to an Australian Merino ram which was sold for $16,000 AUD.

Medium wool breeds have wool between the extremes, and are typically fast-growing meat and ram breeds with dark faces. Some major medium wool breeds, such as the Corriedale, are dual-purpose crosses of long and fine-wooled breeds created for high-production commercial flocks. Long wool breeds are the largest of sheep, with lengthy wool and a slow rate of maturation. Long wool sheep are most valued by modern agriculture for crossbreeding to improve the attributes of other sheep types. The American Columbia breed was developed through crossing Lincoln rams—a long wool breed—with fine-wooled Rambouillet ewes.

Coarse or carpet wool sheep are those with a medium to long length wool of characteristic coarseness. Breeds traditionally used for carpet wool show more variability in general traits than other types, the chief requirement being a wool that will not break down under heavy use (as would that of the finer breeds). As the demand for carpet-quality wool declines, some breeders of this type of sheep are attempting to reposition a few of the traditional breeds to alternative purposes. Others have always been primarily meat-class sheep.

A last group of sheep breeds is that of fur or hair sheep, which do not grow wool at all. Hair sheep are similar to the very early type of domesticated sheep kept before wooly breeds were developed, and are primarily raised for meat and pelts. Some modern breeds of hair sheep, such as the Dorper, are the result of crosses between wooled and hair breeds. For producers uninterested in selling wool, hair sheep are highly advantageous, as those who keep hair sheep need not go to the expense of shearing. Hair sheep are also resistant to parasites and hot weather, and are consequently increasing in popularity among a subset of producers.

With the modern rise of corporate agrobusiness and the decline of localized family farms, many breeds of sheep are in danger of extinction. Preference for only those breeds with uniform characteristics and fast growth rates has pushed heritage (or heirloom) breeds to the margins of the sheep industry. Those that remain are maintained through the efforts of conservation organizations, breed registries, and individual farmers dedicated to their preservation.

GENETIC IMPROVEMENT OF DAIRY CATTLE

Dairymen are constantly concerned with improvement of their herds. Dairy cattle improvement is expressed most frequently as increased milk production and less often in terms of changes in body conformation or "type." Improvement in milk production can be considered as being environmental or genetic. Both environmental and genetic factors contribute to variation in milk production. There are environmental and genetic limitations of production. More importantly, management of environment and genetic factors can result in improved performance, i.e., greater milk production.

Genetic Principles of Repeatability

Understanding the concept and knowing the repeatability of economically important traits help considerably in deciding which cows to cull. Repeatability also is important in sire proofs. All repeatability estimates represent some type of correlation. The trait one is considering, and the times and places it was measured, influence the estimate.

The correlation between 305-day mature equivalent milk records of first-calf heifers, and their records as second-calf heifers, is about 0.5.

So milk records are said to have a repeatability of 0.5. Conception rate from year-to-year with the same cow has a repeatability of about zero, indicating that there is little or no relationship (correlation) between the number of services it takes for a cow to become pregnant each time.

These estimates are useful in making culling and management decisions, since they help us make the best possible guess at how well the cow will do next year if we know how well she did this year. For milk yield, 50 per cent of the apparent superiority (or inferiority) of the cow for this year will appear next year on the average.

If a cow gave 1000 pounds more than her herdmates this year, the best prediction of her yield next year will be 500 pounds more. Naturally, what she actually does is another story; she could be much better or much worse than our guess. The same process is used for below average cows; only one-half of their apparent inferiority will appear the following year on the average. Repeatability is included in the calculation of estimated relative producing ability in DHI.

Only a fraction of the cow's performance is permanent (repeatable). Superior cows may do even better next year, but on the average they do worse; inferior cows on the average do better.

Genetic Principle of Heritability

Heritability is a measure of the degree to which a trait such as milk yield is genetically determined. Although not all of the genetic contribution is included, essentially all which is available to a breeder who is trying to select within a breed is included. Obviously heritability is an important factor among the several factors determining how much genetic improvement can be made in any characteristic.

One of the disadvantages with the dairy cow, in attempts to make genetic progress, is that most of the economically important traits can be measured only in the female. Another disadvantage is that heritabilities are low or close to zero in several cases. A zero heritability would mean that no genetic change could be expected from usual selection techniques.

A practical idea of the meaning of heritability can be obtained easily. A genetically average group of males is mated to a large group of high producing first calf heifers. These heifers average 1000 pounds of milk more than their contemporaries. Assume also that no extraordinary changes in environment have occurred by the time that daughters from these matings freshen and complete their first record.

How much milk will the daughters produce compared to their herdmates? Answer: about 100 to 150 pounds more. Reason: milk yield has a heritability of about 20 to 30 per cent, and since the sires used were genetically average, and sires and dams contribute about equally to the genotype of their offspring, only 10 to 15 per cent of the superiority of the dams will be seen in the offspring.

A good practical definition of heritability is, therefore, the fraction of the merit (or lack of merit) observed in the parents which can be seen in the offspring, with merit being defined as a deviation from the population average.

Note that several reproductive traits have very low heritabilities. Milk yield would be said to be moderately heritable; fat and protein percentages are highly heritable.

One possibility exists for genetic improvement of important traits with zero or very low heritability. This revolves around what geneticists call nonadditive genetic variance.

If there is appreciable nonadditive genetic variance, it can be taken advantage of by crossbreeding. Heterosis (hybrid vigour) is a reflection of this type of genetic variability. Unfortunately, although there is some heterosis in reproductive performance, longevity, livability and milk yield, it is not a large amount.

Crossbreeding has several disadvantages for dairy cattle, although this discussion cannot be covered here. Few people are ready to advise taking advantage of nonadditive genetic variance in dairy cattle at the present time, and few cattleman are attempting to do so. Reproductive efficiency can be improved considerably by improving management practices while selection is being practiced for more highly heritable traits.

SELECTION AND EXPECTED RESPONSE

Traits which are heritable presumably can be changed by selection, but the degree of heritability is only one of three factors which determine the progress which can be made. The other two are the culling level (intensity of selection) and the variability of the trait. These are logical since the more severely we can cull, the more progress we can make. Also, the more variable a trait is, the higher the population average will be for the selected individuals for any given culling percentage.

It turns out that the amount of progress which can be made in one generation is the product of intensity of selection, heritability for that trait, and the observed variability. Note that if any of the three components is zero, selection progress will be zero also.

Good estimates are available for how much progress can be made from selection for most of the economically important characteristics of dairy cattle. Of course, there are several traits which are important, so there is a need to look further than anticipated results from selection for a single trait.

Correlated Response

Knowing what the genetic relationships are among the important traits, plus a few other things, permits us to predict what will happen to a trait such as fat percentage if we ignore it completely and select for milk yield, or vice versa. Though these results pertain to Holsteins, they are similar to results for other breeds.

The changes expected in the trait being selected for; values off the diagonal are changes expected to happen in other traits. Heritabilities and variabilities used in these calculations agreed with those generally accepted by dairy cattle geneticists. Intensity of selection in the estimations was fairly conservative. If more severe culling were practiced, greater progress would be made.

If milk yield alone is selected for at a reasonable level of intensity, an increase is expected in genetic merit in the next generation of 607 pounds. Since milk yield, fat yield and protein yield are genetically fairly closely related (that is, their genetic correlations are high and positive), an increase is expected in fat and protein yields, even though these were ignored in the selection programme.

Because of the negative genetic correlations between milk yield and fat percentage, and milk yield and protein percentage, these two percentages are expected to go down. Selecting for milk yield and ignoring the other four traits would be expected to result in an increase per generation of 607 pounds of milk, 23.2 pounds of fat and 13.7 pounds of protein, but decreases of 0.036 per cent fat and 0.018 per cent protein.

If one attempted to increase fat percentage genetically in his herd by selecting for it and ignoring other traits, he could increase fat percentage. A reasonable increase per generation to be expected is 0.190 per cent. Along with this, however, there would be an actual decrease in milk yield of 287 pounds, although fat yield would increase 24.1 pounds.

Present pricing systems for milk in the United States are based mostly on its weight and fat percentage, although additional factors such as protein percentage may be included also. So the dairyman needs to decide what combination of milk yield and fat percentage and other changes is most profitable for him. He also needs to produce milk that passes minimum legal standards; this is an important factor in herds which already are near the minimum. Beyond this, there are a number of other important traits which must be considered. Dairymen, of course, mentally put all of these factors together in their selection programmes and, depending on their present herd status and present milk pricing, give each trait a certain amount of emphasis.

In other words, they weight each characteristic they think is important. Geneticists do the same thing and attempt to establish numerical values for the weights; a numerical index, called a selection index, then can be formulated for each economic situation.

Milk Yield and Composition

Just about every index formulated for the United States gives yield more emphasis than any other trait, with enough emphasis placed on fat percentage to meet legal standards. Protein has become more important in pricing systems in recent years.

Reproductive Performance

Efficient reproduction is very important economically because a cow must first reproduce to produce. However, most measures of heritability are zero or close to zero, suggesting that little or no improvement can be made by selection. There already is considerable selection pressure being exerted on improving reproductive performance without any conscious effort being made by the breeder. This occurs because sterile males and females leave no offspring, and those with low efficiency leave a lot fewer than those of higher reproductive performance.

So within a given herd culling for reproductive failure would have little effect on the genetic merit for reproduction of the herd. Now that large numbers of records are being obtained on reproduction of daughters of AI sires, however, it may turn out that this information can be taken advantage of in selecting which proven AI sires to use in the herd. Even though heritability of most single measures of reproduction are close to zero, estimates of average genetic merit of a large group of daughters for reproductive efficiency are much more reliable.

Desirable Body Type

Desirable type has appealed to dairymen for centuries, and major changes in appearance in dairy cattle have occurred over the years, accompanied by increases in milk yield. This fact does not itself mean that the two traits have (or ever have had) an appreciable, positive genetic correlation. Regardless of what has gone before, the breeder must concern himself with the present facts of life in his selection programme.

The genetic relationship between type and production seems close to zero and may even be negative. There have been a number of changes in the breed association type classification programmes and policies in recent years, and evaluation of all such changes cannot yet be made. A number of scoring systems also have been developed by others such as universities and AI studs. Yet the final value of desirable type must be in its relationship with production and longevity of the cow.

Except for the breeder who derives an important fraction of his income from sale of breeding stock, dairymen should realise (according to research) that only 2 to 6 per cent of their income is related to variability in body confirmation. USDA researchers estimated several years ago that giving equal emphasis to type and production would reduce the possible increase in milk yield by 29 per cent. Though perhaps the final judgment on emphasis to be placed on desirable type cannot yet be made, it appears that if major attempts are made to improve type, they will be made at the sacrifice of possible genetic increases in milk yield.

Longevity

Longevity may be defined as the ability to avoid death or

culling, the former being mostly for disease or accident and the latter for reproductive failure, low milk yield, mastitis, etc. Few cows die simply from old age. Of the various possible reasons for loss, some have a genetic basis but few are highly heritable.

In any event, high producing cows remain in the herd longer than low producers. Natural selection pressures also work in favour of the ability to resist death or culling. Selection for high milk yield, plus natural selection, seem to be exerting sufficient selection pressure for increased longevity such that the breeder need not give it major emphasis in his programme.

Body Size and Weight

Within each dairy breed, large cows give more milk, on the average, than small cows, but they also require more feed. Research suggests that the additional costs involved with larger cows about equal the additional income derived from them. In the case of two cows of equal production but different size, one actually would expect the smaller cow to be more profitable. Most measures of size (weight, height, etc.) show appreciable heritability and variability, so larger cows could doubtless be developed if desired.

However, most research now suggests that milk yield in dairy cows can be increased considerably without there being any increase in size. Selection for increased body size could be successful, but the correlated response in milk yield though probably positive would be close to zero. Though North Carolina researchers indicated that it might still be wise to check cows considerably above or below the breed average in body weight for productivity and longevity, they concluded that "undue emphasis on larger cows in the short run could lead to the development of less profitable animals."

Other Traits

Many others are economically important and are heritable to some degree. Many qualitative (simply inherited) traits, ranging from lethals on one extreme to aesthetic traits on the other, can be important under some circumstances. Artificial insemination, particularly frozen semen, has caused concern because of possible widespread dissemination of undesirable genes. The genetics of the situation have been studied, however, and with present knowledge potential dangers apparently can be avoided.

Traits other than those mentioned also are important. Mastitis resistance, is of extreme economic value and has measurable heritability. A certain amount of direct pressure for resistance will be exerted from culling of mastitic animals, although clinical cases may remain in a dairy herd for years under proper treatment.

Present knowledge of genetics of dairy cattle suggests that major selection emphasis should be placed on milk yield, with enough selection pressure on fat percentage to maintain composition of milk at legal standards. Other components of milk may become important if pricing systems change to emphasize them.

Care should be taken to include as few traits as practical in a selection programme, since progress in milk yield may be sacrificed to a degree such that total profit per cow may decrease. This is especially true with traits of low heritability and only slight genetic relationship to milk yield. Reproductive efficiency and resistance to mastitis may appear as economically important traits in future sire proving systems.

The Animal Model

The Animal Model does many things notably different from previous evaluation systems. These include simultaneous evaluation of all sires and cows.

This means all information on all relatives is used to increase the accuracy of any one animal's evaluation. This also means that cow families are directly included in the evaluation of all sires and cows, effectively eliminating the basis for previous objections by some breeders. All female ancestors and descendants are used in the evaluation of both sires and cows, weighted by how closely they are related. Since all known relatives of both registered and grade cows are used, computing the evaluations for the Holstein breed requires simultaneous solution of about 50 million equations. Other changes include correction for genetic merit of mates, use of a new genetic base, new ways of using records on cows missing first records and cows changing herds, and definition of different management groups for registered and grade cows.

There is some new terminology with the Animal Model emphasizing that new methods are truly different.

Predicted Difference (PD) changes to Predicted Transmitting Ability (PTA), or one-half the breeding value. This is the prediction of what the sire transmits to his offspring. Cow Index changes to Predicted Transmitting Ability (PTA).

Repeatability (RPT) changes to reliability. Repeatability always has been a misnomer as used by the USDA in this context anyway. Since reliability includes contributions from additional relatives, reliability figures should be higher than the old repeatabilities. The biggest difference is for sires of cows with few daughters compared to those with many. A sire with no daughters would have a reliability of 37 per cent.

Percentile is sire's ranking based on the active AI bull population; for cows it will be based on cows with recent lactations. The rankings are based on an index including milk, fat, and protein evaluations. Previously they were based on an index including only milk and fat.

As good as the new Animal Model system is, it cannot correct for preferential treatment of daughters of certain sires. No genetic evaluation system can. Random AI sampling of young sires and wide daughter distribution will continue to be important in establishing accurate first evaluations. This also is true for sires with relatively few daughters.

Economic Evaluation of Sires and Their Semen

Predicted transmitting ability for dollar value (PTA PRO$) is based on milk, fat, and protein evaluations. Current national prices are used. For the July 1989 run these were $11.20 per hundredweight of milk containing 3.5 per cent milk fat and 3.2 per cent protein. Hence the equation for estimating PTA PRO$ is PTA PRO$ = $.0242 (PTA milk) + $ 1.54 (PTA fat) + $ 1.09 (PTA protein). Note that the dollar value is computed from pounds fat and protein produced, not percentages. Percentile rankings are based on this index.

In Florida, the milk price is higher than almost everywhere else in the United States, and the dollar values of superior sires should be proportionally higher. The ranking of bulls by evaluations would not change much, but the net value over their semen price would.

Taking advantage of considerable previous research, Marsha Wilcox and coworkers developed techniques to aid dairymen in the selection of semen to purchase for herd use. The concept is that of net present value (discounted net income) of semen.

Although the method is computationally elaborate, availability of microcomputers to dairymen will permit each to develop a system of evaluating semen based on a set of selection criteria tailored to individual needs. Information necessary for semen selection include sire proof for milk, fat, protein, type (PDT), interest rate, and such management parameters for the individual herd as conception rate, calving interval and female mortality rate.

Outcome of this linear net merit index for semen is Present Value Dollars (PV$). These researchers then evaluated a number of possible economic and management situations to determine the effects on sire selection; considerable shifting of rank occurred with changes in criteria.

For one sample selection programme (all selection pressure on milk, none on desirable type), rank correlations of PV$ and PDM, and PV$ and PD$ + semen price, were.56 and.52. Such procedures should prove useful and profitable to dairymen who are able to characterize their own management parameters and to define their selection goals. Thus, the concepts of proving sires are not difficult. Efforts to obtain better estimates, thus increasing rates of genetic improvement, continue to make the exact calculations and formulas very complex.

SELECTING SIRES FOR A SINGLE HERD

Most of the factors involved in sire selection have been

covered in earlier sections, but one major question remains. Will the sire which has been proven to be superior in other herds also be superior in my herd? Older breeders will remember the term "nicking," which is not too often heard anymore. If a sire did well in one herd and poorly in a second, he was said to nick well in the first, poorly in the second.

Today, researchers look at the importance of nicking by studying the importance of sire by farm interactions. Such interactions arise if there are real changes in the relative performance of sires (usually measured by the milk yield of their daughters) as they are used on various farms. Should there be an appreciable number of sires which rank high in some herds or farms, and low in others, and vice versa for other sires, this would show up as a sire-by-herd interaction.

The importance of this question is apparent; if there were such interactions, a dairymen would be unable to rely on USDA sire proofs, since he could not depend on sires with superior proofs to be superior in his herd. This was an area that obviously needed research, and during the past several years considerable research has been published on the subject.

A classic study by North Carolina scientists involved sire-by-region interactions. The two regions involved were North Central and Southeastern United States and the question essentially was, "Do AI sires used in these two areas rank about the same, or are there some who are outstanding in one region but poor in the other, and vice versa?" Much of the semen used by Florida dairymen is from sires bred, house and proven in the Eastern and North Central United States, so this question was of immediate concern.

Results showed that this particular type of interaction was not an important factor, and indeed was almost nonexistent. The authors stated, "provided adequate unbiased progeny information is utilized, a bull may be safely selected and used for artificial insemination in one region, even though he was evaluated in the other region."

Studies on the importance of sire by herd interactions have been in very close agreement, with one being conducted by Florida researchers on records of Florida DHIA Guernsey,

Holstein and Jersey first-calf heifers. Everyone recognizes that even the best bull may have a certain number of poor daughters and that a dairyman who has only a few daughters of a particular sire may have been unlucky, by chance, and gotten one or more of them. The opposite can happen also with poor sires. The problem is to determine how important the interactions are overall, realizing that a certain amount of shifting in rankings of sires can occur by chance, particularly if a sire is represented in one or more herds by only a small number of daughters.

The research found that under Florida DHIA herd conditions; these interactions were of little or no practical or theoretical consequence for milk and fat yields. There was some evidence among Guernsey's and Jerseys of an interaction for fat percentage; this has been suggested in other research studies also, but many of the scientists who have studied interactions have not looked at fat percentage.

In summary, it appears that sires proven superior for milk and fat yields in other herds can be used with confidence in Florida dairy herds, without concern for possible sire by herd interactions. The possibility exists for the presence of interactions with fat percentage.

FINDING SUPERIOR FEMALES

Measurements for most of the economically important traits can be made directly on females. It frequently takes a long time to get the measurements of interest, however. Mature body size, would have to wait until the cow is 6 to 8 years old. An estimate of milk yield must wait until the first lactation is completed (at about 3 years of age), unless one accepts an estimate of the lactation based on the first several months.

These points are mentioned because genetic progress is influenced by the time at which measurements are made, and their reliability. Take milk yield as an example. An estimate of the milk producing ability of a cow comes with her first milk record. Certainly, however, one knows more about her when there are two records rather than one, and even more with three records. Generally, the more records available, the more reliable the estimate of her real ability; but it takes longer to get more records. An estimate of the producing ability of a cow was called "Most Probable Producing Ability" years ago by Dr. J.L. Lush, well known animal geneticist. This measure takes into consideration the idea of repeatability, and shows how the number of records a cow has should influence the estimate of her producing ability. If a heifer produces more than her herdmates during her first lactation, we will certainly guess that she is a better than average animal.

If the average of her first two records is above herdmates, one would be even more confident that she is truly above average, and her good performance did not just happen from some favourable accident which probably will not happen again.

The calculations are simple and can be applied to any trait of interest. Although the concept is rarely mentioned today, since availablity of computers makes more sophisticated procedures feasible, MPPA serves as the basis for modern methods. State the milk record, or any other measurement, as a deviation from herdmates. If the cow has two measurements, state each as a deviation, and take the average. MPPA then can be calculated as:

MPPA = (Average deviation) × [(nr)/(1 + nr – r)]

where n = the number of measurements and r = the repeatability. How much better two measurements or records are than one, as far as reliability, is determined by a similar equation.

Gain in accuracy = 1 – [(1 + nr – r) / n]

with n and r as in MPPA. The more records one has on a cow, the more one can accept her records at face value. If she has six records averaging 2000 pounds better than her herdmates, the best guess of her MPPA is 1714 pounds better.

Which cow should be selected as a dam for a future herd sire, a cow with two records averaging 3000 pounds above herdmates, or one with four records averaging 2400 pounds above? The two estimates of MPPA are close, being 2000 pounds for the cow with two records and 1920 pounds for the older cow. One probably would look at other characteristics of the two animals, particularly fat percent but possibly others, before making a decision. The more sophisticated and useful application of this concept, of course, is that it is incorporated into calculations of ERPA.

GENETIC CHANGE IN MILK YIELD

The theoretical upper limits of genetic change in milk yield have been known for quite some time. Knowing the various repeatabilities, heritabilities, generation intervals and selection pressures (intensities), one can calculate what would be expected to happen. This tells nothing about what is actually going on, of course, but it does tell what one can expect under the best conditions.

Potential

If milk yield is given maximum emphasis in the selection programme, with little or no pressure being exerted on other traits, and efficient use is made of an AI sire proving programme, the maximum attainable genetic change in milk yield is slightly over 2.0 per cent per year. Most of this, over 90 per cent, theoretically would come directly or indirectly from sire selection. In a Holstein population averaging 15,000 pounds per cow, this would amount to 300 pounds per year. Though this estimate has appeared disappointingly small to some breeders, it is more than the actual total change which has been attained in the United States.

Observed

It is only in recent years that it has been possible to obtain reliable estimates of the actual genetic change which has occurred in milk production. A major problem in the actual measurement of such progress is that environmental and genetic changes are confounded in such a manner over time as to make their separation extremely difficult. With the availability of high-speed large-capacity electronic computers, many of the problems can now be handled. Use of the animal model has improved the accuracy of the estimates.

As far as progress arising from selection of males and

females, theoretical estimates has been right on target. About 90 to 92 per cent of all genetic change in milk yield has occurred from sire selection; this represents the selection of males and females to produce herd sires and the selection of males to produce herd dams. The remaining 8 to 10 per cent of genetic progress arises from selection of females to produce herd dams. The fact that we must raise nearly all female calves born alive in a population to maintain population size, and the difficulties of evaluating the true genetic merit of dams, precludes much selection pressure from selection of dams.

Average annual genetic change in milk yield of tested dairy cattle has been variable but seems to be about 0.7 per cent of their average levels. This would amount to about 105 pounds per cow in a 15,000 pound herd, or 140 pounds in a 20,000 pound herd. In individual herds, one would expect to find genetic changes which were considerably higher or lower. If 2.0 per cent annual genetic change is possible, as theory suggests, dairymen are progressing genetically only about one-third as fast as possible.

DOG

The dog is a domesticated subspecies of the wolf, a mammal of the Canidae family of the order Carnivora. The term encompasses both feral and pet varieties and is also sometimes used to describe wild canids of other subspecies or species. The domestic dog has been one of the most widely-kept working and companion animals in human history, as well as being a food source in some cultures. There are estimated to be 400,000,000 dogs in the world.

The dog has developed into hundreds of varied breeds. Height measured to the withers ranges from a few inches in the Chihuahua to a few feet in the Irish Wolfhound; colour varies from white through grays to black, and browns from light to dark in a wide variation of patterns; and, coats can be very short to many centimeters long, from coarse hair to something akin to wool, straight or curly, or smooth.

In breeding circles, a male canine is referred to as a *dog,* while a female canine is called a *bitch*. The father of a litter is called the *sire,* and the mother of a litter is called the *dam*. Offspring are generally called *pups* or *puppies* until they are about a year old. A group of offspring is a *litter*. The process of birth is *whelping*. Many terms are used for dogs that are not purebred.

Origin and Evolution

Based on DNA evidence, the wolf ancestors of modern dogs diverged from other wolves about 100,000 years ago, and dogs were domesticated from those wolf ancestors about 15,000 years ago. This date would make dogs the first species to be domesticated by humans.

Evidence suggests that dogs were first domesticated in East Asia, possibly China, and some of the peoples who entered North America took dogs with them from Asia.

As humans migrated around the planet a variety of dog forms migrated with them. The agricultural revolution and subsequent urban revolution led to an increase in the dog population and a demand for specialization. These circumstances would provide the opportunity for selective breeding to create specialized working dogs and pets.

This ancient mosaic, likely Roman, shows a large dog with a collar hunting a lion. Molecular systematics indicate that the domestic dog descends from one or more populations of wild wolves. As reflected in the nomenclature, dogs are descended from the wolf and are able to interbreed with wolves.

The relationship between human and canine has deep roots. Converging archaeological and genetic evidence indicate a time of domestication in the late Upper Paleolithic close to the Pleistocene/Holocene boundary, between 17,000 and 14,000 years ago. Fossil bone morphologies and genetic analysis of current and ancient dog and wolf populations have not yet been able to conclusively determine whether all dogs descend from a single domestication event, or whether dogs were domesticated independently in more than one location. Domesticated dogs may have interbred with local populations of wild wolves on several occasions (a process known in genetics as introgression).

The earliest dog fossils, two crania from Russia and a mandible from Germany, date from 13,000 to 17,000 years ago. Their likely ancestor is the large northern Holarctic wolf, *Canis lupus lupus*. Remains of smaller dogs from Mesolithic cave deposits in the Middle East, dated to around 12,000 years ago, have been interpreted as descendants of a lighter Southwest Asian wolf, *Canis lupus arabs*.

Rock art and skeletal remains indicate that by 14,000 years ago, dogs were present from North Africa across Eurasia to North America. Dog burials at the Mesolithic cemetery of Svaerdborg in Denmark suggest that in ancient Europe dogs were valued companions.

Genetic analyses have so far yielded divergent results. The ancestors of dogs split off from other wolves between 75,000 and 135,000 years ago, while a subsequent analysis indicated a "common origin from a single gene pool for all dog populations" between 40,000 and 15,000 years ago in East Asia.

Both sets of dates must be reevaluated in light of recent findings showing that poorly calibrated molecular clocks have systematically overestimated the age of geologically recent events. On balance, and in agreement with the archaeological evidence, 15,000 years ago is the most likely time for the wolf-dog divergence.

Development of Dog Breeds

Dogs have been bred into a variety of shapes, colours and sizes. Variation can be wide even within a breed, as with these Cavalier King Charles Spaniels.

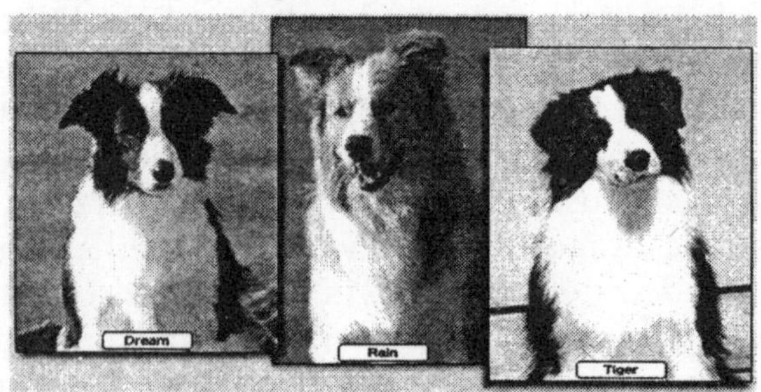

Fig. Dog Breed

There are numerous dog breeds, with over 800 being recognized by various kennel clubs worldwide. Many dogs, especially outside the United States of America and Western Europe, belong to no recognized breed. A few basic breed types have evolved gradually during the domesticated dog's relationship with humans over the last 10,000 or more years, but all modern breeds are of relatively recent derivation. Many of these are the product of a deliberate process of artificial selection. Because of this, some breeds are highly specialized, and there is extraordinary morphological diversity across different breeds. Despite these differences, dogs are able to distinguish dogs from other kinds of animal.

The definition of a dog breed is a matter of some controversy. Depending on the size of the original founding population, closed gene pool breeds can have problems with inbreeding, specifically due to the founder effect. Dog breeders are increasingly aware of the importance of population genetics and of maintaining diverse gene pools. Health testing and new DNA tests can help avoid problems, by providing a replacement for natural selection. Without selection, inbreeding and closed gene pools can increase the risk of severe health or behavioural problems.

Some organizations define a breed more loosely, such that an individual may be considered of one breed as long as 75 per cent of its parentage is of that breed. These considerations affect both pets and the show dogs entered in dog shows. Even prize-winning purebred dogs sometimes possess crippling genetic defects due to founder effect or inbreeding. These problems are not limited to purebred dogs and can affect cross-breed populations. The behaviour and appearance of a dog of a particular breed can be predicted to a degree, while mixed-breed dogs show a broader range of innovative appearance and behaviour.

Mixed-breed dogs or Mongrels (also called "mutts") are dogs that do not belong to specific breeds, being mixtures more than two in variant percentages. Mixed breed dogs and purebred dogs are both suitable as companions, pets, working dogs, or competitors in dog sports. Sometimes different breed dogs are deliberately bred, to create cross-breeds such as the Cockapoo, a mixture of Cocker Spaniel and Miniature Poodle.

Such deliberate crosses may display some degree of hybrid vigour and other desirable traits, but may or may not inherit any of the desired traits of their parents, such as temperament or a particular colour or coat. Without genetic testing of the parents, the crosses can end up inheriting genetic defects that occur in both parental breeds.

A breed is a group of animals that possesses a set of inherited characteristics that distinguishes it from other animals within the same species. Deliberately crossing two or more breeds is also a manner of establishing new breeds, but it is only a breed when offspring will reliably demonstrate that particular set of characteristics and qualities.

Breed Popularity

Breed popularity varies widely over time and in different parts of the world and different segments of the population. Counting by American Kennel Club (AKC) registration (not by licensing registration or by United Kennel Club (UKC) registration, which could present different statistics), the Labrador Retriever has been the United States's most commonly registered breed of dog since 1991.

However, even within parts of the United States, popularity varies; for example, in 2005 the most-registered breed in New York City was the Poodle while the Yorkshire Terrier was the second-most-registered breed in Houston. However, animal shelters in many parts of the United States report that the most-commonly available dog for adoption is the American Pit Bull Terrier or pit bull-type mixes, making up as much as 20 per cent of dogs available for adoption, none of which would be registered with the AKC. Two decades ago, in 1983, the AKC's top two registered breeds were the American Cocker Spaniel and the Poodle.

In the United Kingdom, The Kennel Club reports that the most-registered breed from at least 1999 to 2005 was the Labrador Retriever. It rounds out the top three for 1999 to 2005 with the German Shepherd Dog, also popular in the States, and the English Cocker Spaniel, which is no longer even in the top ten in the States. In the United Kingdom a national dog adoption and rescue service indicates that the most common breed appearing in shelters is the Greyhound followed by the Staffordshire Bull Terrier.

Physical Characteristics

Modern dog breeds show more variation in size, appearance, and behaviour than any other domestic animal. Within the range of extremes, dogs generally share attributes with their wild ancestors, the wolves. Dogs are predators and scavengers, possessing sharp teeth and strong jaws for attacking, holding, and tearing their food.

Although selective breeding has changed the appearance of many breeds, all dogs retain basic traits from their distant ancestors. Like many other predatory mammals, the dog has powerful muscles, fused wristbones, a cardiovascular system that supports both sprinting and endurance, and teeth for catching and tearing. Compared to the bone structure of the human foot, technically, dogs walk on their toes.

Differences from Other Canids

Compared to equally sized wolves, dogs tend to have 20 per cent smaller skulls and 10 per cent smaller brains, as well as proportionately smaller teeth than other canid species. Dogs require less calories to function than wolves. Their diet of human refuse in antiquity made the large brains and jaw muscles needed for hunting unnecessary. It is thought by certain experts that the dog's limp ears are a result of atrophy of the jaw muscles. Dogs tend to be poorer than wolves and coyotes at observational learning, being more responsive to instrumental conditioning.

Dogs have thicker skins than similairly sized wolves. Inuits tend to favour dog skin over wolf skin due to the formers resistance to tear. Unlike wolves, but like coyotes, domestic dogs have sweat glands on their pawpads. The paws of a dog are half the size of those of a wolf, and their tails tend to curl upwards, another trait not found in wolves. Feral dogs show little of the complex social structure or dominance heirarchy present in wolf packs. For dogs, other members of their kind are of no help in locating food items, and are more like competitors. Dogs differ from wolves and most other large canid species by the fact that they do not regurgitate food for their young, nor the young of other dogs in the same territory.

Many dogs, such as this American Water Spaniel, have had their natural hunting instincts suppressed or altered to suit human needs. Like most mammals, dogs are dichromats and have colour vision equivalent to red-green colour blindness in humans. Different breeds of dogs have different eye shapes and dimensions, and they also have different retina configurations.

Dogs with long noses have a *"visual streak"* which runs across the width of the retina and gives them a very wide field of excellent vision, while those with short noses have an *"area centralis"*—a central patch with up to three times the density of nerve endings as the *visual streak*—giving them detailed sight much more like a human's.

Some breeds, particularly the sighthounds, have a field of vision up to 270° (compared to 180° for humans), although broad-headed breeds with short noses have a much narrower field of vision, as low as 180°.

Dogs detect sounds as low as the 16 to 20 Hz frequency range (compared to 20 to 70 Hz for humans) and above 45 kHz (compared to 13 to 20 kHz for humans), and in addition have a degree of ear mobility that helps them to rapidly pinpoint the exact location of a sound. Eighteen or more muscles can tilt, rotate and raise or lower a dog's ear. Additionally, a dog can identify a sound's location much faster than a human can, as well as hear sounds up to four times the distance that humans are able to. Those with more natural ear shapes, like those of wild canids like the fox, generally hear better than those with the floppier ears of many domesticated species.

Dogs have nearly 220 million smell-sensitive cells over an area about the size of a pocket handkerchief (compared to 5 million over an area the size of a postage stamp for humans). Some breeds have been selectively bred for excellence in detecting scents, even compared to their canine brethren. What information a dog actually detects when he is scenting is not perfectly understood; although once a matter of debate, it now seems to be well established that dogs can distinguish two different types of scents when trailing, an air scent from some person or thing that has recently passed by, as well as a ground scent that remains detectable for a much longer period.

The characteristics and behaviour of these two types of scent trail would seem, after some thought, to be quite different, the air scent being intermittent but perhaps less obscured by competing scents, whereas the ground scent would be relatively permanent with respect to careful and repetitive search by the dog, but would seem to be much more contaminated with other scents.

In any event, it is established by those who train tracking dogs that it is impossible to teach the dog how to track any better than it does naturally; the object instead is to motivate it properly, and teach it to maintain focus on a single track and ignore any others that might otherwise seem of greater interest to an untrained dog. An intensive search for a scent, for instance searching a ship for contraband, can actually be very fatiguing for a dog, and the dog must be motivated to continue this hard work for a long period of time.

Domestic dogs often display the remnants of countershading, a common natural camouflage pattern. The general theory of countershading is that an animal that is lit from above will appear lighter on its upper half and darker on its lower half where it will usually be in its own shade. This is a pattern that predators can learn to watch for. A countershaded animal will have dark colouring on its upper surfaces and light colouring below.

This reduces the general visibility of the animal. One reminder of this pattern is that many breeds will have the occasional "blaze", stripe, or "star" of white fur on their chest or undersides.

Dogs can generate large amounts of energy for a short period of time. A dog's heart and lungs are oversized relative to its body and its normal everyday needs. A dog also has relatively more red blood cells than a human. Most of the time the dog will keep the extra red blood cells stored in its spleen. When the animal enters into a situation where its full metabolism is required, such as play, catching game, or fighting other dogs, the extra cells are released into the bloodstream.

The "oversized" heart and lungs will now be running at full capacity, and the animal will have an enhanced ability to engage in aerobic activity. This activity will produce internal heating. Dogs, being covered in fur, are limited in their ability to cool down. After a short time the animal must either cease its athletic activity or risk harming itself from overheating. One can easily observe this pattern of intense activity followed by rest periods in puppies. During the rest phase the spleen collects red blood cells and the animal may pant to cool down.

Dogs are very social animals, but their personality and behaviour vary with breed as well as how they are treated by their owners and others who come in contact with them. It is not uncommon for dogs to attack humans and other animals; however, this is usually because of lack of care or improper upbringing by its owner.

Many dogs can be trained to skillfully perform tasks not natural to canines, such as in this dog agility competition.

Dogs are valued for their intelligence. This intelligence is expressed differently with different breeds and individuals, however. For example, Border Collies are noted for their ability to learn commands, while other breeds may not be so motivated towards obedience, but instead show their cleverness in devising ways to steal food or escape from a yard. Being highly adaptable animals themselves, dogs have learned to do many jobs as required by humans over the generations.

Dogs are employed in various roles across the globe, proving invaluable assets in areas such as search-and-rescue; law enforcement (including attack dogs, sniffer dogs and tracking dogs); guards for livestock, people or property; herding; Arctic exploration sled-pullers; guiding the blind and acting as a pair of ears for the deaf; assisting with hunting, and a great many other roles which they may be trained to assume. Most dogs rarely have to deal with complex tasks and are unlikely to learn relatively complicated activities (such as opening doors) unaided. Some dogs (such as guide dogs for the visually impaired) are specially trained to recognize and avoid dangerous situations.

The meaning of "intelligence" in general, not only in reference to dogs, is hard to define. Some tests measure problem-solving abilities and others test the ability to learn in comparison to others of the same age. Defining it for dogs is just as difficult. It is likely that dogs do not have the ability to premeditate an action to solve a problem.

For example, the ability to learn quickly could be a sign of intelligence. Conversely it could be interpreted as a sign of a desire to please. In contrast, some dogs who do not learn very quickly may have other talents. An example is breeds that are not particularly interested in pleasing their owners, such as Siberian Huskies. Huskies are often fascinated with the myriad of possibilities for escaping from yards, catching small animals, and often figuring out on their own numerous inventive ways of doing both.

Assistance dogs are also required to be obedient at all times. This means they must learn a tremendous number of commands, understand how to act in a large variety of situations, and recognize threats to their human companion, some of which they might never before have encountered. Many owners of livestock guardian breeds believe that breeds like the Great Pyrenees or the Kuvasz are not easily trained because their stubborn nature prevents them from seeing the point of such commands as "sit" or "down".

Hounds may also suffer from this type of ranking. These dogs are bred to have more of a "pack" mentality with other dogs and less reliance on a master's direct commands. While they may not have the same kind of intelligence as a Border Collie, they were not bred to learn and obey commands quickly, but to think for themselves while trailing game.

Dogs are highly social animals. This can account for their trainability, playfulness, and ability to fit into human households and social situations. These attributes have earned dogs a unique position in the realm of interspecies relationships despite being one of the most effective, voracious, and potentially dangerous predators. Dogs and humans at times co-operate in some of the most effective hunting in the animal world; in that context, dogs are superpredators.

The loyalty and devotion that dogs demonstrate as part of their natural instincts as pack animals closely mimics the human idea of love and friendship, leading many dog owners to view their pets as full-fledged family members. Conversely, dogs seem to view their human companions as members of their pack, and make few, if any, distinctions between their owners and fellow dogs. Dogs fill a variety of roles in human society and are often trained as working dogs. For dogs that do not have traditional jobs, a wide range of dog sports provide the opportunity to exhibit their natural skills. In many countries, the most common and perhaps most important role of dogs is as companions.

Dogs have lived and worked with humans in so many roles that their loyalty has earned them the unique sobriquet "man's best friend". However, some cultures consider dogs to be unclean. In some parts of the world, dogs are raised as livestock to produce dog meat for human consumption. In many places, consumption of dog meat is discouraged by social convention or cultural taboo.

Laughter might not be confined or unique to humans, despite Aristotle's observation that "only the human animal laughs". The differences between chimpanzee and human laughter may be the result of the adaptations that enable human speech. However, some behavioural psychologists argue that self-awareness of one's situation, or the ability to identify with somebody else's predicament, are prerequisites for laughter, so animals are not really laughing in the same way that humans do.

The dog-laugh sounds similar to a normal pant. However by analyzing the pant using a spectrograph, this pant varies with bursts of frequencies, resulting in a laugh. When this recorded dog-laugh vocalization is played to dogs in a shelter setting, it can initiate play, promote pro-social behaviour, and decrease stress levels. In a study by Simonet, Versteeg, and Storie, one hundred and twenty subject dogs residing in a mid-size county animal shelter were observed. Dogs ranging from 4 months to 10 years of age were compared with and without exposure to a dog-laugh recording.

The stress behaviours measured included panting, growling, salivating, pacing, barking, cowering, lunging, play-bows, sitting, orienting and lying down. The study resulted in positive findings.

Exposure to the dog laughing recording resulted in the following: significantly reduced stress behaviours, increased tail wagging and the display of a play-face when playing was initiated, and more frequent pro-social behaviour such as approaching and lip licking. This research suggests exposure to dog-laugh vocalizations can calm and possibly increase shelter adoptions.

HORSE BREEDING

Horse breeding refers to reproduction in horses, and particularly the human-directed process of selective breeding of animals, particularly purebred horses of a given breed. While feral and wild horses breed successfully without human assistance, planned matings can be used to produce specifically desired characteristics in domesticated horses. Furthermore, modern breeding management and technologies can increase the rate of conception, a healthy pregnancy, and successful foaling.

The male parent of a horse, a stallion, is commonly known as the sire and the female parent, the mare, is called the dam. Both are genetically important, as each parent provides half of the genetic makeup of the ensuing offspring, called a foal. (Contrary to popular misuse, the word "colt" refers to a young male horse only; "filly" is a young female.)

Though many amateur horse owners may simply breed a family mare to a local stallion in order to produce a companion animal, most professional breeders use selective breeding to produce individuals of a given phenotype, or breed. Alternatively, a breeder could, using individuals of differing phenotypes, create a new breed with specific characteristics. Some breeders consider the quality of the sire to be more important than the quality of the dam. However, other breeders maintain that the mare is the most important parent. Because stallions can produce far more offspring than mares, a single stallion can have a greater overall impact on a breed. However, the mare may have a greater influence on an individual foal because its physical characteristics influence the developing foal in the womb and the foal also learns habits from its dam when young.

Foals may also learn the "language of intimidation and submission" from their dam, and this imprinting may affect the foal's status and rank within the herd. Many times, a mature horse will achieve status in a herd similar to that of its dam; the offspring of dominant mares become dominant themselves.

Estrus Cycle of the Mare

The estrous cycle controls when a mare is sexually receptive toward a stallion, and helps to physically prepare the mare for conception. It generally occurs during the spring and summer months, although some mares may be sexually receptive into the late fall, and is controlled by the photoperiod (length of the day), the cycle first triggered when the days begin to lengthen. The estrus cycle lasts about 19-22 days, with the average being 21 days. As the days shorten, the mare returns to a period when she is not sexually receptive, known as anestrus. Anestrus prevents the mare from conceiving in the winter months, as that would result in her foaling during the harshest part of the year, a time when it would be most difficult for the foal to survive. This cycle contains 2 phases:

- Estrus, or Follicular, phase: 5-7 days in length, when the mare is sexually recepetive to a stallion. Estrogen is secreted by the follicle. Ovulation occurs in the final 24-48 hours of estrus.
- Diestrus, or Luteal, phase: 14-15 days in length, the mare is not sexually recepetive to the stallion. The corpus luteum secretes progesterone.

Although 16 per cent of mares have double ovulations (allowing them to twin), this does not affect the length of time of estrus or diestrus.

Effects on the Reproductive System During the Estrous Cycle

Changes in hormone levels can have great affects on the physical characteristics of the reproductive organs of the mare, thereby preparing, or preventing, her from conceiving.

- Uterus: increased levels of estrogen cause edema within the uterus, making it feel heavier, and the uterus loses its tone. This edema decreases following ovulation, and the muscular tone increases. High levels of progesterone do not cause edema within the uterus. The uterus becomes flaccid during anestrus.
- Cervix: the cervix relaxes right before estrus occurs, and the secretions of the cervix increase. High progesterone levels (during diestrus) cause the cervix to close.
- Vagina: the portion of the vagina near the cervix becomes engorged with blood right before estrus. The vagina becomes relaxed and secretions increase.
- Vulva: relaxes right before estrus begins. Becomes dry, and closes tightly, during diestrus.

Hormones Involved in the Estrus Cycle, During Foaling, and after Birth

The cycle is controlled by several hormones which regulate the estrous cycle, the mare's behaviour, and the reproductive system of the mare. The cycle begins when the increased day length causes the pineal gland to reduce the levels of melatonin, thereby allowing the hypothalamus to secrete GnRH.

- *GnRH (Gonadotropin releasing hormone):* Secreted by the hypothalamus, causes the pituitary to release of 2 gonadotrophins: LH and FSH.
- *LH (Luteinizing hormone):* Levels are highest 2 days following ovulation, then slowly decrease over 4-5

days, dipping to their lowest levels 5-16 days after ovulation. Stimulates the follicle to develop, which in turn causes an increase in estrogen. Unlike most mammals, the mare does not have an increase of LH right before ovulation.

- *FSH (Follicle-stimulating hormone):* Secreted by the pituitary, causes the ovarian follicle to develop. Levels of FSH rise slightly at the end of estrus, but have their highest peak about 10 days before the next ovulation. FSH is inhibited by inhibin, at the same time LH and estrogen levels rise, which prevents immature follicles from continuing their growth.
- *Estrogen:* Secreted by the developing follicle, it causes the pituitary gland to secrete more LH (therefore, these 2 hormones are in a positive feedback loop). Additionally, it causes behavioural changes in the mare, making her more recpetive toward the stallion, and causes physical changes in the cervix, uterus, and vagina to prepare the mare for conception. Estrogen peaks 1-2 days before ovulation, and decreases within 2 days following ovulation.
- *Inhibin:* Secreted by the developed follicle right before ovulation, "turns off" FSH, which is no longer needed now that the follicle is larger.
- Progesterone: Prevents conception and decreases sexual receptibility of the mare to the stallion. Progesterone is therefore lowest during the estrus phase, and increases during diestrus. It decreases about 15 days after ovulation, when the corpus luteum begns to decrease in size.
- Prostaglandin: Secreted by the endrometrium 13-15 days following ovulation, causes luteolysis and prevents the corpus luteum from secreting progesterone
- eCG (equine chorionic gonadotropin - formerly called PMS/PMSG pregnant mare serum and pregnant mare serum gonadotropin): Chorionic gonadotropins secreted if the mare conceives. First secreted by the

endometrial cups around the 36th day of gestation, peaking around day 60, and decreasing after about 120 days of gestation. Also help to stimulate the growth of the fetal gonads.

- *Prolactin*: Stimulates lactation
- *Oxytocin*: Stimulates the uterus to contract

While horses in the wild mate and foal in mid to late spring, many horses domestically bred for competitive purposes, especially horse racing and various futurities, are usually born as close to January first as possible, so as to be at an advantage in size and maturity when competing against other horses in the same age group. When an early foal is desired, barn managers will put the mare "under lights" by keeping the barn lights on in the winter to simulate a longer day, thus bringing the mare into estrus sooner than she would in nature.

Mares signal estrus and ovulation by urination in the presence of a stallion, raising the tail and revealing the vulva. A stallion, approaching with a high head, will usually nicker, nip and nudge the mare, as well as sniff her urine to determine her readiness for mating.

Once fertilized, the oocyte (egg) remains in the oviduct for approximately 5.5 more days, and then descends into the uterus. The initial single cell combination is already dividing and by the time of entry into the uterus, the egg might have already reached the blastocyst stage.

The gestation period lasts for about eleven months, or about 342 days (normal average range 320-370 days). During the early days of pregnancy, the embryo (up to about 35 days), or fetus (after 35-40 days), is mobile, moving about in the uterus until about day 16 when "fixation" occurs. True implantation - invasion into the endometrium of any sort - does not occur until about day 35 of pregnancy with the formation of the endometrial cups, and true placentation (formation of the placenta) is not initiated until about day 40-45 and not completed until about 140 days of pregnancy.

A heartbeat can be detected on day 21, and the fetus gender can be determined by day 70 of the gestation. Halfway through gestation the fetus is the size of between a rabbit and a beagle. The most dramatic fetus development occurs in the last 3 months of pregnancy when 60 per cent of fetal growth occurs.

Care of the Pregnant Mare

Domestic mares receive specific care and nutrition to ensure that they and their foals are healthy. Mares are given vaccinations against diseases such as the Rhinopneumonitis (EHV-1) virus (which can cause abortions) as well as vaccines for other conditions that may occur in a given region of the world.

Mares can be used for riding or driving during most of their pregnancy, and it's healthy for them to have exercise. But only moderate exercise, especially when they become heavy in foal. Exercise in excessively high temperatures has been suggested as being detrimental to pregnancy maintenance during the embryonic period - it should however be noted that ambient temperatures encountered during the research were in the region of 100 degrees F and the same results may not be encountered in regions with lower ambient temperatures.

Mares are generally fed more than other horses and are provided supplemental vitamins and minerals because their bodies require extra nutrition to form (and later to nurse) a foal. Many feeds designed for pregnant and lactating mares also have extra fat and protein. Overfeeding the pregnant mare should also be avoided, as excess weight may contribute to difficulties foaling or fetal/foal related problems.

A special foaling stall or shed that is large and clutter free provides the mare with a safe place to give birth. Most mares foal at night or early in the morning, and prefer to give birth alone when possible. Labour is rapid, often no more than 30 minutes, and from the time the feet of the foal appear to full delivery is often only about 15 to 20 minutes. Once the foal is born, the mare will lick the newborn foal to clean it and help blood circulation. In a very short time, the foal will attempt to stand and get milk from its mother. A foal should stand and nurse within the first hour of life.

To create a bond with her foal, the mare licks and nuzzles the foal, enabling her to distinguish hers from others. Some mares are aggressive when protecting their foals, and may attack other horses or unfamiliar humans that come near their newborns.

After birth, a foal's navel is dipped in iodine to prevent infection, it is sometimes given an enema to help clear the meconium from its digestive tract, and the newborn is monitored to ensure that it stands and nurses without difficulty. While most horse births happen without complications, many owners have first aid supplies prepared and a veterinarian on call in case of a birthing emergency.

People who supervise foaling should also watch the mare to be sure that she passes the placenta in a timely fashion, and that it is complete with no fragments remaining in the uterus, where they could cause a serious infection. If the placenta is not removed from the stall after it is passed, a mare will often eat it, an instinct from the wild, where blood would attract predators.

Foals develop rapidly, and within a few hours a wild foal can travel with the herd. In domestic breeding, the foal & dam are usually kept separate for a while, but within a few weeks are typically pastured with the other horses. A foal will begin to eat hay, grass & grain alongside the mare at about 4 weeks old; by 10-12 weeks the foal requires more nutrition than the mare's milk can supply. Foals are typically weaned at 4-8 months of age, although in the wild a foal may nurse for a year.

How Breeds Develop

Beyond the appearance and conformation of a specific type of horse, breeders aspire to improve physical performance abilities. This concept, known as matching "form to function," has led to the development of not only different breeds, but also families or bloodlines within breeds that are specialists for excelling at specific tasks.

For example, the Arabian horse of the desert naturally developed speed and endurance to travel long distances and survive in a harsh environment, and domestication by humans added a trainable disposition to the animal's natural abilities. In the meantime, in northern Europe, the locally adapted heavy horse with a thick, warm coat was domesticated and put to work as a farm animal that could pull a plow or wagon. This animal was later adapted through selective breeding to create a strong but ridable animal suitable for the heavily-armored knight in warfare.

Then, centuries later, when people in Europe wanted faster horses than could be produced from local horses through simple selective breeding, they imported Arabians and other oriental horses to breed as an outcross to the heavier, local animals. This led to the development of breeds such as the Thoroughbred, a horse taller than the Arabian and faster over the distances of a few miles required of a European race horse or light cavalry horse. Another cross between oriental and European horses produced the Andalusian, a horse developed in Spain that was powerfully built, but extremely nimble and capable of the quick bursts of speed over short distances necessary for certain types of combat as well as for tasks such as bullfighting.

Later, the people who settled the Americas needed a hardy horse that was capable of working with cattle. Thus, Arabians and Thoroughbreds were crossed on Spanish horses, both domesticated animals descended from those brought over by the Conquistadors, and feral horses such as the Mustangs, descended from the Spanish horse, but adapted by natural selection to the ecology and climate of the west. These crosses ultimately produced new breeds such as the American quarter horse and the Criollo of Argentina.

In modern times, these breeds themselves have since been selectively bred to further specialize at certain tasks. One example of this is the American quarter horse. Once a general-purpose working ranch horse, different bloodlines now specialize in different events. For example, larger, heavier animals with a very steady attitude are bred to give competitors an advantage in events such as team roping, where a horse has to start and stop quickly, but also must calmly hold a full-grown steer at the end of a rope. On the other hand, for an event known as cutting, where the horse must separate a cow from a herd and prevent it from rejoining the group, the best horses are smaller, quick, alert, athletic and highly trainable. They must learn quickly, have conformation that allows quick stops and fast, low turns, and the best competitors have a certain amount of independent mental ability to anticipate and counter the movement of a cow, popularly known as "cow sense."

Another example is the Thoroughbred. While most representatives of this breed are bred for horse racing, there are also specialized bloodlines suitable as show hunters or show jumpers. The hunter must have a tall, smooth build that allows it to trot and canter smoothly and efficiently. Instead of speed, value is placed on appearance and upon giving the equestrian a comfortable ride, with natural jumping ability that shows bascule and good form.

A show jumper, however, is bred less for overall form and more for power over tall fences, along with speed, scope, and agility. This favours a horse with a good galloping stride, powerful hindquarters that can change speed or direction easily, plus a good shoulder angle and length of neck. A jumper has a more powerful build than either the hunter or the racehorse. The history of horse breeding goes back millennia. Though the precise date is in dispute, humans could have domesticated the horse as far back as approximately 4500 BCE. However, evidence of planned breeding has a more blurry history.

One of the earliest people known to document the breedings of their horses were the Bedouin of the Middle East, the breeders of the Arabian horse. While it is difficult to determine how far back the Bedouin passed on pedigree information via an oral tradition, there were written pedigrees of Arabian horses by A.D. 1330. The Akhal-Teke of West-Central Asia is another breed with roots in ancient times that was also bred specifically for war and racing. The nomads of the Mongolian steppes bred horses for several thousand years as well.

The types of horses bred varied with culture and with the times. The uses to which a horse was put also determined its qualities, including smooth amblers for riding, fast horses for carrying messengers, heavy horses for plowing and pulling heavy wagons, ponies for hauling cars of ore from mines, packhorses, carriage horses and many others.

Medieval Europe bred large horses specifically for war, called destriers. These horses were the ancestors of the great heavy horses of today, and their size was preferred not simply because of the weight of the armor, but also because a large horse provided more power for the knight's lance. Weighing almost twice as much as a normal riding horse, the destrier was a powerful weapon in battle.

On the other hand, during this same time, lighter horses were bred in northern Africa and the Middle East by Muslim warriors, who preferred a faster, more agile horse. The lighter horse suited the raids and battles of the Bedouins, allowing them to outmaneuver rather than overpower the enemy. When Muslim warriors and European knights collided in warfare, the heavy knights were frequently outmaneuvered.

The Europeans, however, soon made up for the lack of speed of their native breeds by incorporating genetic traits from captured oriental horses such as the Arabian, Barb to their stables. This cross-breeding led both to a nimbler war horse, such as today's Percheron, but also to created a type of horse known as a Courser, a predecessor to the Thoroughbred, which was used as a message horse.

During the Renaissance, horses were bred not only for war, but for haute ecole riding, derived from the most athletic movements required of a war horse, and popular among the elite nobility of the time. Breeds such as the Lipizzan were developed from Spanish-bred horses for this purpose, and also became the preferred mounts of cavalry officers, who were derived mostly from the ranks of the nobility.

It was during this time that gunpowder was developed, and so the light cavalry horse, a faster and quicker war horse, was bred for a "shoot and run" tactic rather than the close hand-to-hand fighting seen in the Middle Ages. After Charles

II retook the British throne in 1660, horse racing, which had been banned by Cromwell, was revived. The Thoroughbred was developed 40 years later, bred to be the ultimate racehorse, through the lines of 3 foundation Arabian stallions.

The 17th and 18th centuries saw more of a need for fine carriage horses in Europe, bringing in the dawn of the warmblood. The warmblood breeds have been exceptionally good at adapting to changing times, and from their carriage horse beginnings they easily transitioned during the 1900s into a sport horse type. Today's warmblood breeds, although still used for competitive driving, are more often seen competing in the show jumping or dressage arenas. The Thoroughbred continues to dominate the horseracing world, although its lines have been more recently used to improve warmblood breeds and to develop sport horses.

The predecessor of the American Quarter Horse was developed in the 1700s, mainly for quarter racing (racing ¼ of a mile). The breed was later adapted for work in the west, and "cow sense" was particularly bred for as their use for herding cattle increased. However, because there was also a need for animals suitable for sprint racing, the modern Quarter Horse has two distinct types: the sleeker racing type and the stock horse type. The racing type most resembles the finer-boned ancestors of the first racing Quarter Horses, and the type is still used for ¼-mile races. The stock horse type, used in western events, is bred for a shorter stride, docile temperament, and cow sense.

The need for horses for heavy draft and carriage work continued until the industrial revolution and the advent of the automobile and the tractor. After this time, draft and carriage horse numbers dropped significantly, though light riding horses remained popular for recreational pursuits. Draft horses today are used on a few small farms, but today are seen mainly for pulling and plowing competitions rather than farm work. Heavy harness horses are now used as an outcross with lighter breeds, such as the Thoroughbred, to produce the modern warmblood breeds popular in Olympic and sport horse disciplines.

Breeding a horse is an endeavor where the owner, particularly of the mare, will usually need to invest considerable time and money. For this reason, a horse owner needs to consider several factors, including:

- Does the proposed breeding animal have valuable genetic qualities to pass on?
- Is the proposed breeding animal in good physical health, fertile, and able to withstand the vigors of reproduction?
- For what purpose will the foal be used?
- Is there a market for the foal in the event that the owner does not wish to keep the foal for its entire life?
- What is the anticipated economic benefit, if any, to the owner of the ensuing foal?
- What is the anticipated economic benefit, if any, to the owner(s) of the sire and dam or the foal?
- Does the owner of the mare have the expertise to properly manage the mare through gestation and parturition?
- Does the owner of the potential foal have the expertise to properly manage and train a young animal once it is born?

There are value judgements involved in considering whether an animal is suitable breeding stock, hotly debated by breeders. Additional personal beliefs may come into play when considering a suitable level of care for the mare and ensuing foal, the potential market or use for the foal, and other tangible and intangible benefits to the owner.

If the breeding endeavor is intended to make a profit, there are additional market factors to consider, which may vary considerably from year to year, from breed to breed, and by region of the world. In many cases, the low end of the market is saturated with horses, and the law of supply and demand thus allows little or no profit to be made from breeding unregistered animals or animals of poor quality, even if registered.

The minimum cost of breeding for a mare owner includes

the stud fee, and the cost of proper nutrition, management and veterinary care of the mare throughout gestation, parturition, and care of both mare and foal up to the time of weaning. Veterinary expenses may be higher if specialized reproductive technologies are used or health complications occur. Making a profit in horse breeding is often difficult. While some owners of only a few horses may keep a foal for purely personal enjoyment, many individuals breed horses in hopes of making some money in the process.

A general rule of thumb is that a foal intended for sale should be worth three times the cost of the stud fee if it were sold at the moment of birth. From birth forward, the costs of care and training are added to the value of the foal, with a sale price going up accordingly. If the foal wins awards in some form of competition, that may also enhance the price.On the other hand, without careful thought, foals bred without a potential market for them may wind up being sold at a loss, and in a worst-case scenario, sold for "salvage" value — a euphemism for sale to slaughter as horsemeat.

Therefore, a mare owner must consider their reasons for breeding, asking hard questions of themselves as to whether their motivations are based on either emotion or profit and how realistic those motivations may be.The stallion should be chosen to complement the mare, with the goal of producing a foal that has the best qualities of both animals, yet avoids having the weaker qualities of either parent. Generally, the stallion should have proven himself in the discipline or sport the mare owner wishes for the "career" of the ensuing foal. Mares should also have a competition record showing that they also have suitable traits, though this does not happen as often.

A purebred horse is usually worth more than a horse of mixed breeding, though this matters more in some disciplines than others. The breed of the horse is sometimes secondary when breeding for a sport horse, but some disciplines may prefer a certain breed or a specific phenotype of horse. Sometimes, purebred bloodlines are an absolute requirement: For example most Racehorses in the United States must be recorded with a breed registry in order to race. Bloodlines are often considered, as some bloodlines are known to cross well with others. If the parents have not yet proven themselves by competition or by producing quality offspring, the bloodlines of the horse are often a good indicator of quality and possible strengths and weaknesses.

Some bloodlines are known not only for their athletic ability, but could also carry a conformational or genetic defect, poor temperament, or for a medical problem. Some bloodlines are also fashionable or otherwise marketable, which is an important consideration should the mare owner wish to sell the foal. Horse breeders also consider conformation, size and temperament.

All of these traits are heritable, and will determine if the foal will be a success in its chosen discipline. The offspring, or "get," of a stallion are often excellent indicators of his ability to pass on his characteristics, and the particular traits he actually passes on. Some stallions are fantastic performers but never produce offspring of comparable quality.

Others sire fillies of great abilities but not colts. At times, a horse of mediocre ability sires foals of outstanding quality. Mare owners also look into the question of if the stallion is fertile and has successfully "settled" (i.e. impregnated) mares. A stallion may not be able to breed naturally, or old age may decrease his performance. Mare care boarding fees and semen collection fees can be a major cost. Breeding a horse can be an expensive endeavor, whether breeding a backyard competition horse or the next Olympic medalist. Costs may include:

- The stud and booking fee
- Fees for collecting, handling, and transporting semen (if AI is used and semen is shipped)
- Mare exams: to determine if she is healthy enough to breed, to determine when she ovulates, and (if AI is used) to inseminate her
- Mare transport, care, and board if the mare is bred live cover at the stallion's residence
- Veterinary bills to keep the pregnant mare healthy while in foal

- Possible veterinary bills during pregnancy or foaling should something go wrong
- Veterinary bills for the foal for its first exam a few days following foaling

Stud fees are determined by the quality of the stallion, his performance record, the performance record of his get (offspring), as well as the sport and general market that the animal is standing for.

The highest stud fees are generally for racing Thoroughbreds, which may charge from two to three thousand dollars for a breeding to a new or unproven stallion, to several hundred thousand dollars for a breeding to a stakes winner. Sport horse stallions generally range from $1000 to $3000, although the top stallions may reach $4000 for one breeding. The lowest stud fees may only be $100-$200, but there are trade-offs: the horse will probably be unproven, and probably much less athletic than a horse with a stud fee that is a bit higher.

As a stallion's career, either performance or breeding, improves, his stud fee tends to increase in proportion. If one or two offspring are especially successful, winning several stakes races or an Olympic medal, the stud fee will generally greatly increase. Younger, unproven stallions will generally have a lower stud fee earlier on in their careers.

To help decrease the risk of financial loss should the mare die or abort the foal while pregnant, many studs have a live foal guarantee (LFG), allowing the owner to have a free breeding to their stallion the next year. However, this is not offered for every breeding.

Chapter 5

Pathogens to Animals

WAYS PATHOGENS SPREAD

In order to prevent the introduction of pathogens, one must understand how pathogens find their way onto backyard, hobby, and large corporate poultry or livestock operations. The spread of pathogens is primarily caused by the movement of animals, people, and contaminated equipment. Therefore, you can help prevent the spread of pathogens by controlling the movement of people and animals and avoiding contact with any potentially-contaminated equipment or objects.

Controlling Animal Movement and Contact

The easiest and most frequent way to transmit a pathogen is for an infected animal to come into contact with a healthy animal. Most disease is transmitted nose-to-nose or by other direct contact with sick animals. New additions to flocks or herds are a very common way to introduce pathogens. Stray pets that wander onto your farm or land can be another source of pathogen transmission.

If a sick animal is allowed into a show or fair, it may infect other nearby animals. In addition to stray pets; wild animals, free-flying birds, and insects can be responsible for the introduction of a pathogen.

People Movement People, vehicles, equipment, and clothing that are in contact with an infected animal may be contaminated with pathogens. These contaminated articles include equipment, machinery, and other objects used for the transportation, care, and management of livestock and poultry.

If pathogens can be spread from animal to animal at shows and fairs, does that mean that we cannot take an animal to the show? We can purchase animals and go to the fair, but you should isolate those animals when you return. The wisest decision is to choose shows and make livestock and poultry purchases from places where disease prevention is always given high priority.

Practical Steps that Improve Isolation

Isolation (a form of quarantine) prevents contact between animals within a controlled environment. The idea behind isolation is to prevent contact between healthy animals and an animal that is or could be infected with a pathogen. Animals new to the herd or flock should be isolated away from the rest of the herd or flock for at least four weeks. Always isolate sick animals and only return them to their original group when they've fully recovered. Livestock returning from fairs or shows should also be isolated, since they could have picked up a new pathogen at the show.

After returning to the farm, you should isolate your show animals to avoid the possibility of infecting other animals on your farm. Ideally, this should be in a completely separate place to avoid close contact. At minimum it could be a separate pen in a different building or at least a separate corner of the barn. This may represent some extra work, but it can be very important. Isolate all purchased animals for four weeks. If they are incubating a serious disease, the signs (i.e., diarrhea, hard breathing, etc.) of that disease will likely be observed in that 4 week isolation period.

This gives you some time to do follow-up testing or give booster vaccinations if needed. Always purchase good, healthy animals. Do not buy sickly animals, even if they are being sold for a "cheap" price. Livestock or poultry at bargain prices can be expensive!

Since people can carry pathogens on their body or clothing, it is necessary to control the visitors that may come in contact with your livestock or poultry. Always make sure visitors wear clean boots and clothing. It is best if visitors come only when you are there to escort them around your farm. Locked gates and doors will keep people out when you're not around. Signs and notices help to alert visitors of the potential risk that they may pose. Perimeter fences will keep people from accidentally wandering onto your property. Question visitors about the farms or animals they have visited or have been near recently, and ask if they have visited a foreign country within the past 5 days.

There are ways to help keep out wild animals, free-flying birds, and insects. Although it is impossible to totally prevent all contact between wildlife and our livestock, we can make barnyards and surroundings unattractive to many of these species. Cutting the grass and weeds around the outside of buildings will help prevent rodents from entering. Keep grain spills or other potential sources of food cleaned up and unavailable to wildlife.

Clean up old board piles or woodpiles and inspect buildings for possible hiding or denning areas. Inspect the haymow or other protected areas for evidence that cats, raccoons, or other animals that are likely using the hay or the straw for nesting areas. Store feed where wild animals, including rodents and birds, cannot make contact with it. Dispose of all waste feed in a way that will not attract pests. Maintain barns and buildings in good repair making it more difficult for animals or birds to gain access. Keep doors and windows shut when not needed for ventilation. Place screens or netting on the windows.

Location and Construction of Buildings

When planning the location of a barn or building used to house your livestock and/or poultry, isolation is key. The buildings or pens should be constructed to promote isolation from outside sources of disease. The facility should be a substantial distance from road traffic. It is important to consider possible exposure and the distance from other flocks, herds, or populations of domestic or wild animals. It is especially crucial that there is no nose-to-nose or beak-to-beak contact with other animals. There should not be any contact with drainage water or waste runoff from other animals. When planning the organization of either a large- or small-scale animal operation, the risk of disease can be greatly reduced whenever you keep different species and ages of the same species well separated. This is because pathogens producing little or no disease in one species can produce significant disease in another species. Mild infections in older animals can produce severe disease in young animals.Disease susceptibility within the same species varies with age.

Because they have acquired resistance, older animals may shed pathogens without getting sick themselves. These same pathogens can be serious to younger animals. Salmonella and E. coli are good examples of pathogens that can spread and produce extra trouble in young or newborn animals when they are not well separated from older stock.

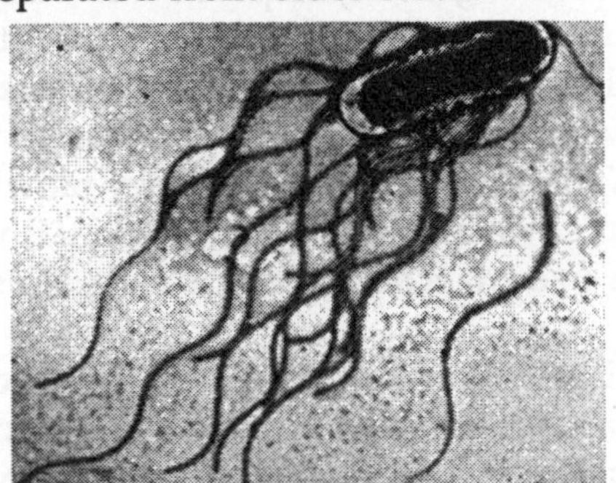

Fig. Salmonella magnified 3000 X

Various ways may be available to achieve species/age separation. They will be different depending on many factors such as the value of the animals, the economic and labour resources available to the herd/flock owner, and such other factors as farm size and marketing opportunities. They may include separate buildings, well-separated pens, different caretakers, or, ideally separate premises for different species and ages. Certain types of farm operations are able to ensure separation of ages by using the "all-in/all-out" management practice. All-in/all-out management allows only one age at a time on a premise. No new or younger animals are brought in until all of the older animals are removed and the barn has been cleaned. This allows for cleaning and disinfecting before a new group of animals is brought onto the premises. The farm environment can be a very comfortable place where pathogens can survive and multiply.

Animal buildings, barns and pastures, as well as litter and manure surfaces, are often damp environments favourable for a dangerous increase in pathogen populations. Depending on the number of animals, very large accumulations of manure and litter may develop and become areas where pathogens can survive and multiply for many weeks or months.

SANITATION

How can you avoid bringing your animals to pathogens? The best way is to maintain a clean, dry, and sanitary environment. Cleaning is very important in reducing pathogen levels. Cleanliness means freedom from dirt, filth, and debris. Although buildings and equipment can appear clean when they are not visibly dirty, many microscopic contaminating pathogens can continue to be present. They remain and survive by clinging to surfaces, and by hiding in tiny cracks and crevices. The use of a disinfectant kills these remaining pathogens

Proper disinfection results in reduction of pathogens. Reducing the amount of pathogens around your animals will decrease the risk of disease. Disinfectants are chemical agents that kill pathogens on contact. However, it is important to clean before disinfecting so that the pathogens become fully exposed to the disinfectant.

Pre-cleaning is doubly important because a disinfectant can be used up or inactivated by dirt. Disinfection and thorough, prompt drying are the last steps in the sanitation process. Without quick, thorough drying, any pathogens surviving the effects of the disinfectant can re-multiply to high numbers.

Hygienic Manure

Animal body wastes (feces, urine, etc.) ordinarily accumulate right in the environment (surroundings) where the animals spend most of their lives. In humans, of course, this does not occur because of toilets, plumbing and sewage treatment/disposal systems. Since flush toilets are not practical for animals, this ordinarily unavoidable problem for animals is partially reduced when manure or litter is managed in a way that, at least lowers the level of exposure to potential pathogens.

Accumulated manure must be managed to reduce its volume, its odor, and to kill pathogens and weed seeds. The essential parts of manure management include collection, transfer, and storage. Spreading manure onto fields is the most common method of disposal.

The sun will dry manure after it is spread onto fields which will kill many pathogens. A proper level of airflow over manure surfaces promotes drying and the decrease of many pathogen populations. In contrast, stagnant air contributes to the build- up of moisture, and an increase in pathogen populations.

Chemical treatments can be beneficial in manure management. Raising the pH to at least 12 for 30 minutes will kill most of the microorganisms present. Lime is usually used to raise the pH. Treatments that produce anaerobic conditions (very low oxygen) are also used. Anaerobic lagoons take advantage of a natural process where manure is digested by beneficial anaerobic bacteria. In contrast, aerobic lagoons add oxygen to the manure.

The addition of oxygen allows more common bacteria to survive and multiply and for the bacteria to break down the waste material. These bacteria convert the manure into carbon dioxide, water, and more beneficial lagoon bacteria. In animal pens or holding areas, we want the bedding and floor dry. Management of areas where water spillage or water accumulation is highest is very important. Good drainage and proper ventilation of buildings will help reduce the dangers of dampness. The frequent removal of wet litter and/or bedding and a continuous, modest flow of air over manure/litter surfaces will help to produce the drying needed to suppress bacteria.

THREATS TO ANIMAL HEALTH FROM THE VISIBLE TO THE INVISIBLE

Animals may be injured or die from the attacks by something as large and dangerous as a coyote or wolf to something just as dangerous, but only as small, as a molecule. This section takes you on a voyage into a world of animal health dangers. This fascinating voyage ranges from dangers that are visible to the naked eye (predators), to some that are more easily seen with a hand lens (internal and external parasites), to some that can only be seen with a microscope (bacteria and viruses).

The voyage continues all the way on down to the sub-microscopic world of disease-producing molecules! More about these visible and invisible hazards to animal health and a short discussion about their prevention is presented below. The discussion is very basic and introductory.

We know that disease-causing pathogens that we cannot see threaten our livestock. In addition, there are also other threats that can be easily seen. Predators may easily be detected; however, many often appear at night or when people are not around. There are ways to help keep out predators that could potentially physically attack and harm your animals.

First, remove all easily accessible food supplies. This may be very difficult depending on the size of the farm and the amount of livestock feed on-hand. Keeping feed bins in good repair and sealed off will help prevent predators from entering areas where feed is stored. Keeping feed bins and feeding areas clean is very important.

An accumulation of waste feed in and around feed bunks attracts animals. A second suggestion is to remove water supplies. This is even more difficult on most farms. Stock tanks often provide a constant water supply and are attractive to predators such as raccoons. Preventing any unnecessary pools of water will help. A third suggestion is to modify habitat and reduce access. Clearing brush and keeping weeds away from barns and buildings will help deter animals just like it will help deter rodents. Finally, you can trap or control predators. There are a variety of traps available to catch animals.

Barns and buildings should be kept in good repair. Predators often enter barns though open doors, or cracks and holes that may exist. Closing doors and patching cracks and holes helps to reduce the problem. Wire mesh or screening on windows can also help.

EXTERNAL PARASITES

Small yet visible threats to livestock include external parasites such as ticks, flies, fleas, lice, mosquitoes, mites, grubs, etc. Parasites are a threat to livestock health just as microbial (invisible) pathogens are a threat. Parasites can transmit and spread microbial pathogens in addition to the harm and damage that they naturally cause by irritating animals and sapping their energy. The most common way to control external parasites is through the use of pesticides or insecticides. Pesticides kill and help control the parasite populations. Pesticides are applied as sprays, dips, pour-ons, dusts, injectables, pastes, boluses, etc. Ear tags impregnated with insecticide are commonly used in cattle.

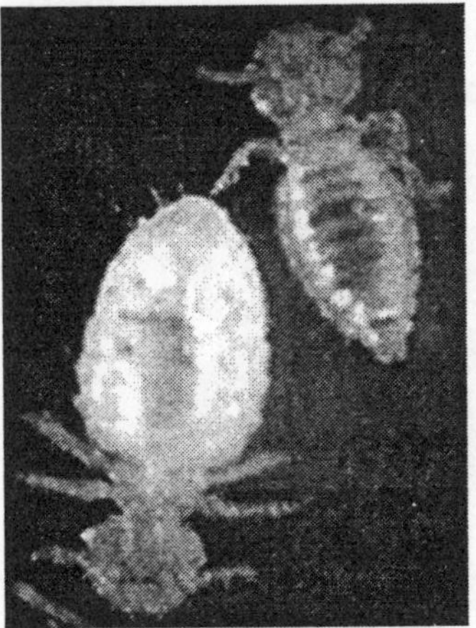

Fig. Lice

Pesticides are very effective however, pesticides alone will not control a threat such as flies. Keeping the environment clean and sanitary helps eliminate fly breeding areas. Manure management will help reduce fly breeding areas. Fly eggs and larvae in thinly spread manure are killed by drying and heat.

INTERNAL PARASITES

Livestock and poultry can be attacked by a variety of large and small worm-like parasites such as roundworms and tapeworms. These internal parasites mainly invade the digestive passages while some also infest an animal's breathing passages. Other parasites can go even deeper into the "donut" or animal body reaching various vital organs and body tissues. Most parasites enter an animal's body when the animal eats the egg (ova) or an early life stage of the parasite.

These ova or intermediate life stages come from the adult parasite reproducing and living inside an animal. They are typically passed by way of animal droppings onto the ground, or into the bedding or litter. As a result, an effective preventive strategy for many internal parasites rests on keeping animals from eating feed or licking surfaces contaminated by animal waste. It is a wise practice to keep animal yards, pens and buildings or other concentration points as clean from urine and accumulated fecal material as is practicable.

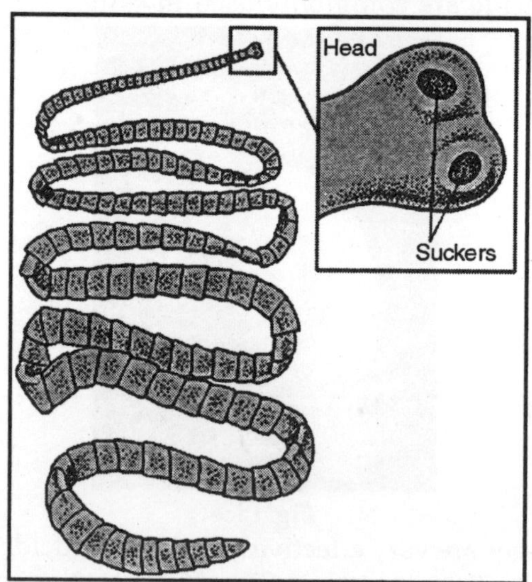

Fig. Tapeworm

Various powerful chemicals are sometimes used to treat different types of infestation. Their improper or inappropriate use may produce more damage to your animals than would be done by the parasites alone. Consequently, it is best to seek guidance from your local veterinarian before you treat for worms. In the final analysis, prevention is often less expensive than treatment.

Bacteria and Viruses

Bacteria and viruses are visible only when they are magnified hundreds to many thousands of times. They are not only able to attack the skin and digestive tract or respiratory linings of an animal's body, but, are often able to devastate the entire body including such organs as the brain, heart, liver and spleen. Their extremely small size makes it possible for these pathogens to survive long periods of times outside an animal's body. They can survive in fur, hair and feathers, in nasal and other discharges from a sick animal, and in animal urine and fecal droppings.

Viruses survive, and bacteria can actually multiply, in animal bedding, litter, and manure. Many survive long periods of time in the tiny particles of dust or soil present in the farm environment. With many tiny, scattered hiding places they can easily be carried to a new farm or group of animals riding on a person's clothing, on the surfaces of boxes, crates or equipment, and on the wheels of cars and trucks. Bacteria are single-celled microorganisms. They may live free in the environment or within a living cell. E. coli (Escherichia coli), Streptococcus, Staphylococcus, and Salmonella are a few examples of bacteria that can cause disease.

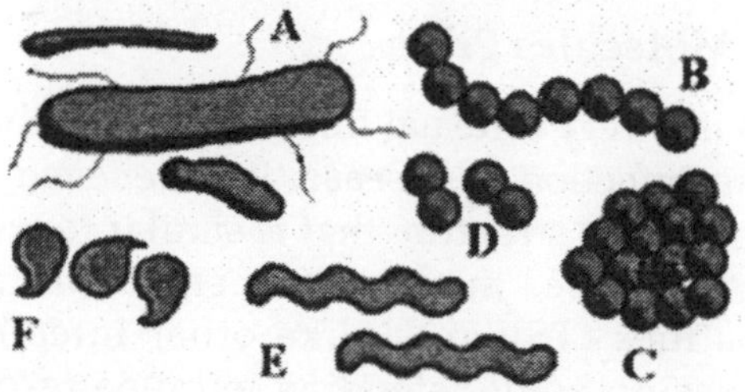

Fig. Bacteria come in a wide variety of shapes: A: Rods; B: Pour ir chains; C: Round in clusters; D: Round in twos; E: Spira; F: Cormma

Viruses are tiny organisms that only grow inside the cells composing the animal's body. All viruses rely on a live animal host to reproduce. Examples of viruses that affect humans include the common cold (rhinovirus) or the flu (influenza) virus. Viruses can infect animals and cause respiratory symptoms (influenza viruses), diarrhea (rotavirus and coronaviruses), and numerous other disorders.

Although common viral or bacterial pathogens are unwelcome visitors or residents, certain ones can be especially troublesome. These special pathogens produce unusually high losses and/or unusual behaviour such as extensive tenderfootedness, incoordination, or slobbering. Milk or egg production may cease or drop sharply. Your daily activities in caring for and feeding your animals put you in an excellent position where you could be among the first to spot the possible emergence of an especially unwelcome pathogen.

As previously emphasized, isolation, traffic control, hygiene, and sanitation are the main ways to keep these essentially invisible pathogens from spreading to, and from reaching levels that can infect your animals! Medications, antibiotics, and vaccines are additional measures available to minimize the effects of bacterial or viral infections. Although powerful allies in an animal's battle with one or more pathogens, they are really the second line of defence.

The first line consists of all the steps you take to keep these microbes out or their numbers down to begin with. Again, those primary steps are herd/flock isolation, traffic control, hygiene, and sanitation.

Dangerous Molecules Prion

A prion is a very unusual infectious agent that is capable of causing an infection or disease. It is believed to be a self-reproducing protein structure that is similar to a virus. Prions cause prion diseases such as transmissible spongiform encephalopathies (TSE's). Unlike other infectious agents, prions produce no body-defending immune response.

Mold Toxins. Mold growth takes place in feeds when they are damp. Mold does not always mean that you cannot use the feed. Most molds are not toxic when fed to livestock; however, some are very toxic. The toxic by-products produced by molds (fungi) are known as mycotoxins (mold toxins). Mold toxins are very diverse because they are produced by many different molds.

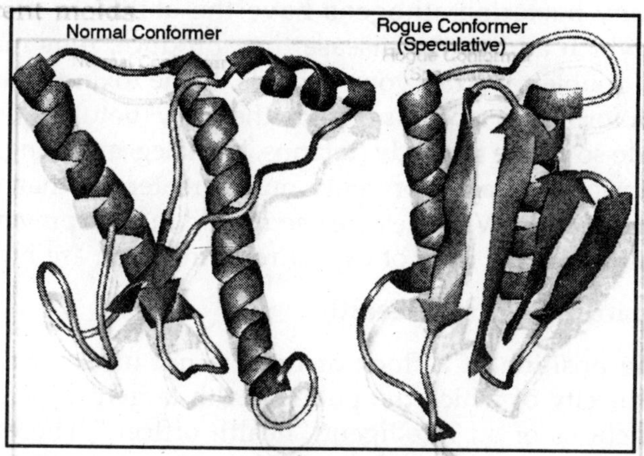

Fig. Prion

Fungi that have the ability to produce mycotoxins are very common in grain and other livestock feeds and in the facilities and equipment used for transportation and storage of feed. They can be very dangerous causing reduced growth rates, lowered immunities, and increased susceptibility to various infectious diseases. Many feed companies are working on ways to sample and test feeds and grains for mold toxins before their sale.

Animals feeds must be kept dry. We must realise that feeding any moldy feedstuffs is a risk to the health of our animal. There is less risk in feeding moldy feeds to fattening animals than for lactating or pregnant animals. The risk is also different among different species of animals.

Dryness is the simplest way to control the growth of mold. Take the following steps when evidence of mold growth (musty odor, visible mold) is suspected.

- Stop the moisture source (fix the leak) correct condensation problems in outside storage bins.
- Thoroughly dry or discard all porous items.

- Scrub mold off hard surfaces with detergent and water, and thoroughly dry. Chlorine-containing products are of help in killing mold spores.

Bacterial Toxins

Many bacterialpathogens have the ability to produce toxins which add to the disease they produce, thus making them a double threat to your animals. Some toxin-producing bacteria form their poisons outside the body (botulism), while others do so inside the body (tetanus, black leg, and gangrene). These toxic bacteria can present a much greater risk than many ordinary bacteria. Vaccines are used to aid in their prevention, particularly where risks of exposure or infection are high.

Safeguarding Animal Health

The position of a flock or herd is not unlike that of a populous city of which the public health largely depends on the functions of an intelligent "health officer." The owner, above all, should function as a health officer to his/her flock or herd. This element of animal management completes the picture of what it takes to keep animals safe and healthy. The health officer idea is especially important to many young people. After all, in the next few years, they may become the owners or managers of even larger populations of animals.

They need to be alert to threats to the health of their own animals, and to those belonging to others. They should be quick to recognize and properly respond to unusual diseases and to oversee and manage their own operations to prevent or minimize the effects of common diseases. The search for and application of disease prevention knowledge can be an enjoyable, enriching lifelong experience. An alert, active disease prevention "mind set" provides many dividends! By protecting your own animals from pathogens you are also helping to protect the animals of others.

ANIMAL DISEASE

The control of animal diseases and the promotion and protection of animal health are essential components of any effective animal breeding and production programme. Despite remarkable technical advances in the diagnosis, prevention and control of animal diseases, the condition of animal health throughout the developing world remains generally poor, causing substantial economic losses and hindering any improvement in livestock productivity.

In developing countries, animal health services were established with the main objective of controlling major contagious and infectious diseases, such as foot-and-mouth disease, rinderpest and contagious pleuropneumonia, as well as parasitic diseases, such as trypanosomiasis and tick-borne diseases. This was obviously the first priority, since the control of these diseases is a prerequisite to any successful livestock development programme.

With the present concern for sustainable economic development, more attention is now being given to other diseases that affect livestock productivity, such as helminthiasis, nutritional diseases, reproductive disorders, etc.

The successful control of disease depends initially on its timely and accurate recognition and on the presence of sound diagnostic capabilities based on effective working links between laboratories and field services. Emergencies created by outbreaks of major infectious diseases demonstrate the need for establishing, strengthening and improving such diagnostic services. As well, particular attention should be given to the development of an efficient animal disease information system.

Beyond the national level, a general increase in the movement of animals and animal products underlines the importance of international cooperation in the prevention and control of animal diseases.

Most animal health services in developing countries do not have at present adequate technical and administrative infrastructures to carry out the tasks and duties necessary for the efficient control of animal diseases and for consumer protection.

In many developing countries, there is either a shortage of skilled veterinary personnel or their services are not correctly utilized. The problem is exacerbated by deficient veterinary infrastructures and inadequate disease control programmes, veterinary legislation and information services, as well as a lack of transport, communications, veterinary products and equipment. The most common problem is the shortage of funds to sustain the activities of veterinary staff. In some developing countries, the animal health services are not given the appropriate legal power in the administrative system.

These shortages significantly reduce the effectiveness of animal health services control measures against major animal diseases. By exploiting existing conditions, local resources and international help, possibilities for improving of animal health service programmes are increased.

Veterinary education and training should receive the highest priority; however, more emphasis must be placed on the qualitative and practical aspects. Effective personnel development requires adequate planning of staff requirements, improved curriculums for undergraduate and postgraduate studies, training of auxiliary personnel and greater interregional cooperation to exploit existing training facilities fully, among other things.

Animal health services should be further developed by improving their efficiency. While the control and prevention of major infectious diseases clearly remains a government responsibility, some veterinary tasks such as the treatment of individual animals could be undertaken in other ways. Privatization is one way of improving some sectors of animal health and of responding suitably to the needs of animal owners.

Other ways include contracting out certain services, creating farmer cooperatives and producer associations, recovering government costs more efficiently and using the revenue thus generated for selective subsidies. Several countries have already taken steps to reorganize their veterinary services in this way.

Developing countries must address this problem. This publication aims to assist them in improving livestock production through better control of major animal diseases. It is not intended to be a comprehensive text describing in-depth all aspects of a complex subject with worldwide variations. Instead, it is meant to serve as a guideline, providing general background information on basic topics. Its main objective is to assist animal health authorities in their organization, planning and management activities.

The contents cover major problems facing official animal health services in developing countries in contributing to the production of food of animal origin and livestock development as integral components of general social, economic and agricultural development. Other priorities of animal health services include the protection of humans against diseases that may be transmitted by animals and the production of safe food.

Biological and pharmaceutical production may be the responsibility of some services, however, only aspects of the control and management of veterinary biologicals and drugs are included in this publication.

The major issues dealt with in this publication are the objectives, functions, organization and management of animal health services. Without going into detail, relevant information, statements and recommendations make up the basic text. This general approach does not permit specific disease control or specific social, economic and ecological conditions to be dealt with. However, information is provided in the annexes on specific topics and in the selected bibliographies of general interest publications.

Chapter 6

Animal Farming

POULTRY FARMING

Commercial raising of chickens, turkeys, ducks, geese, and other birds for their meat and eggs. Since the 1930s and '40s, the poultry industry has become one of the most efficient producers of protein for human consumption. It expanded rapidly during World War II because of the shortage of beef and pork, which require a much longer time to develop; only seven weeks are required to produce a broiler and five months to produce a laying hen.

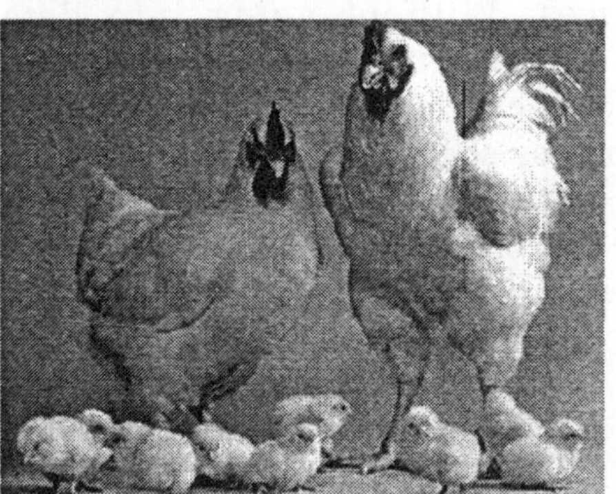

Fig. Poultry Farming.

Between 1980 and 1995, while average U.S. per capita consumption of beef and pork decreased by 11 percent and 6 percent, respectively, consumption of chicken increased by 49 percent and turkey by 74 percent. Concern about dietary cholesterol contributed to a per capita decline in India egg consumption of 14 percent during the same period. India poultry and egg production is federally monitored through the Food Safety and Inspection Service of the India. Department of Agriculture.

Poultry farming is the practice of raising poultry, such as chickens, turkeys, ducks geese, as a subcategory of animal husbandry, for the purpose of farming meat or eggs for food. The vast majority of poultry are farmed using factory farming techniques, 74 percent of the world's poultry meat, and 68 percent of eggs are produced this way.

The contrasting method of poultry farming is free range, and friction between these two main methods has led to long term issues of ethical consumerism. Opponents of factory farming argue that it harms the environment and creates health risks, as well as abusing the animals themselves. In 2002, the United Kingdom also investigated the state of its own poultry farming methods with aims to investigate "animal welfare standards."

The Vegetarian Economy and Green Agriculture (VEGA) research group also states that factory farming of poultry in South-East Asia is a key cause of Avian influenza. However the same has also been said of free-range farming. In return, proponents of factory farming highlight its increased productivity; stating that the animals are looked after in state-of-the-art confinement facilities and are happy; that it is needed to feed the growing global human population; and that it protects the environment.

Chickens

For hundreds of years, chickens were kept in small flocks for home consumption of eggs and meat, with any surplus sold or exchanged for other produce. Not until the 20th century did poultry farming become commercialized. The production of eggs came first; for years the production of broilers was merely an offshoot, the male chickens being raised until 10 to 16 weeks old and then sold for meat.

Today most of the laying hens are housed in wire cages containing from two to ten hens each. The cages may be in a single tier or in tiers of up to five cages. Most of these are automated to provide a constant supply of feed and water and to maintain control of the environment. By comparison with litter floors, where the birds were constantly in contact with one another and with feces, the wire cages increase production efficiency, reduce the incidence of disease, and help keep costs down. A modern poultry farm may have several hundred thousand or even more than a million laying hens.

The Indian. poultry industry comprises somewhat fewer than 300 million such hens, but with modern production techniques they are supplying the nation with more eggs than did a larger hen population some years ago. A dozen eggs can be produced with less than 1.8 kg (less than 4 lb) of feed. Whereas egg-producing hens once produced about 100 eggs each year, such hens can now produce an average of more than 250 eggs each year.

In the mid-1990s the worldwide population of chickens was estimated at 12.7 billion. The annual production of hen eggs exceeded 41.5 million metric tons; China produced about 30 percent of the total. The U.S. is also a leader of the worldwide poultry industry, supplying more than 10 percent of the total egg output. Within the U.S., California produced nearly 9 percent of the nation's 74.3 billion eggs, followed by Ohio, Pennsylvania, Indiana, Georgia, and Iowa.

The modern broiler industry started on a commercial scale on the Delmarva (Delaware-Maryland-Virginia) Peninsula and then spread farther south and southwest. By the mid-1990s the industry was producing more than 7 billion broilers a year, most of them in the southern U.S., with an efficiency such that one unit weight of broiler was being produced with fewer than two unit weights of feed. Nearly all broilers are now the offspring of white Plymouth Rock females and dominant white Cornish males. The leading broiler-producing states are Arkansas, Georgia, Alabama, and North Carolina.

Turkeys

The turkey industry began to develop on a larger scale in the late 1930s and early '40s and has since grown rapidly. At first the birds were grown on ranges, but disease problems forced farmers to raise them on slats or wire platforms. This proved costly and labour inefficient, so when controls were found for the diseases, turkey farms returned to the use of ranges or large houses. In the mid-1990s more than 300 million turkeys were annually produced in the U.S.; North Carolina, Minnesota, Arkansas, California, Virginia, and Missouri were the leading states.

Ducks

Commercially raised ducks numbered about 715 million in the mid-1990s, with China accounting for about 65 percent of the total. The highly specialized duck industry was once concentrated almost entirely in Suffolk Co. on Long Island, N.Y., where more than 10 million ducks were grown each year in the 1960s. Since then, the industry has spread to Indiana and other states.

Ducks are often started at one end of their house and moved along progressively until they are ready for market at approximately seven weeks of age, when they weigh about 3.1 kg. Usually they are started in wire cages and progress to litter floors and outside runs at three to four weeks of age.

Geese

The most geese are produced in small farm flocks of up to a few hundred; few large operations exist. The birds are hardy and are usually grown on ranges, where they are good foragers and require little care after the first two or three weeks. Goose and goose livers remain specialty foods, but the demand for goose down has increased in recent decades. The birds themselves are sometimes used by farmers for weed control.

Free Range

Free range poultry farming consists of poultry permitted to roam freely instead of being contained in any manner. The principle is to allow the animals as much freedom as possible, to live out their instinctual behaviours in a reasonably natural way, regardless of whether or not they are eventually killed for meat.

Unlike in the United States, this definition also applies to eggs. The European Union regulates marketing standards for egg farming which specifies a minimum condition for Free Range Eggs states that "hens have continuous daytime access to open-air runs, except in the case of temporary restrictions imposed by veterinary authorities".

Yarding

While often confused with free range farming, yarding is actually a separate method by which a hutch and fenced off area outside are combined when farming poultry. The distinction is that free-range poultry are either totally unfenced, or the fence is so distant that it has little influence on their freedom of movement.

This is common technique used by small farms in the Northeastern portion of the US. Daily releases out of hutches or coops allow for instinctuial nature for the chickens with protections from predators. The hens usually lay eggs either on the ground of the coop or in baskets if provided by the farmer.

This technique can be complicated if used with roosters though, mostly because of difficulty getting them into the coop and to clean the coop while it is inside. This territorial nature is apparent while outside in which they have a brood of hens and sometimes even informal land claims. This can endanger people unaware of the existence of the territories who are attacked by the larger birds.

Factory Farming

In factory (also known as battery) poultry farming, particularly for eggs, birds are kept in rows of cages, with their environment, ventilation; heating and lighting are dictated automatically.

Extra lighting can be added beyond normal daylight hours to facilitate more egg production, and extra hormones and growth stimulants are added to the feed to encourage egg production or weight gain depending on whether the birds are being farmed for eggs or meat.

ADVANTAGES AND DISADVANTAGES

Free Range

Advantages

Free range poultry farming has the advantage of enabling the poultry to move around, foraging for their natural diet and living in cleaner conditions than in battery farming. In some farms, the manure from free range poultry can be used to benefit crops.

Disadvantages

The practical construction of a free range poultry farm can present more problems than the battery alternative. Finding suitable land with adequate drainage to minimise worms and coocidial oocysts, suitable protection from prevailing winds, good ventilation, access and protection from predators can be difficult. Excess heat, cold or damp can have a harmful effect on the animals and their productivity. Unlike battery farms, free range farmers have little control over the food their animals come across which can lead to unreliable productivity.

Free range farming in the UK, which accounts for 26 per cent of production, has come under similar criticism as battery farming in terms of animal welfare. This is due to the social abnormalities of having large numbers of birds in an outdoor space. Beak trimming due to cannibalism and infighting is common in this form of poultry farming as well as in batteries. Diseases are common and the animals are vulnerable to predators. In South-East Asia, a lack of disease control in free range farming has been associated with outbreaks of avian influenza.

Factory Farming

Advantages

The small cages restrict movement, and allow for more birds per unit area, and this allows for greater productivity and lower space and food costs, with more efforts put into egg laying. Battery farming is quicker, more economical and practical, and growth and output can be specifically controlled. The poultry are at less risk from predators and outdoor elements such as cold, heat, wind or damp, all of which can have significant impact on yield and health of the animals.

Disadvantages

The small environments reduce stimulation of the poultry, which often results in pecking each other or themselves whereas in the outdoors they would have other stimulation. A study by the Agricultural and Food Research Council in 1992 also found that 50 per cent of battery farmed poultry had bone disorders such as osteoporosisor breakages. Battery farms are also at greater risk of fire, due to the amount of electrical equipment and the likelihood of rodents chewing through the wiring. Battery farming is also the subject of much criticism and the products are often less popular than free-range alternatives, and the mislabling of one as the other has led to outrage in some consumer groups.

The use of gas to kill the birdsprior to harvesting was also criticized by Dr. Mohan Raj of United Poultry Concern who stated that current use of carbon dioxide fails to cleanly kill the birds, causing a "a painfully slow death of suffocation" VEGA states that "millions" of male chicks are killed in this way as they do not produce eggs. Debeaking is also heavily criticised due to the psychological effects and pain involved. The act of forced staravtion to reduce periods of off-lay is also unpopular.

Health concerns are not limited to the animals in battery farming, however. The US Department of Health released a list of risks to humans working in poultry battery farms and those living nearby, which included respiratory illnesses and musculoskeletal injuries, infections, odors and flies and chemical and infectious compounds in the soil which included the mixtures of antibodies, pathogens, nutrients, pesticides, hormones and other chemicals that are found in or are administered to battery poultry.

Trace elements of copper or arsenic were also found. Outbreaks of Avian influenza have also been blamed on battery farming in South-East Asia. Battery farming is prohibited in a number of countries, including Switzerland and Sweden, with movements in favour of banning active in the United Kingdom, Australia and Denmark.

AQUACULTURE

FISH FARMING

Fish farming is the principal form of aquaculture, while other methods may fall under mariculture. It involves raising fish commercially in tanks or enclosures, usually for food. A facility that releases juvenile fish into the wild for recreational fishing or to supplement a species' natural numbers is generally referred to as a fish hatchery. Fish species raised by fish farms include salmon, catfish, tilapia, cod, carp, trout and others.

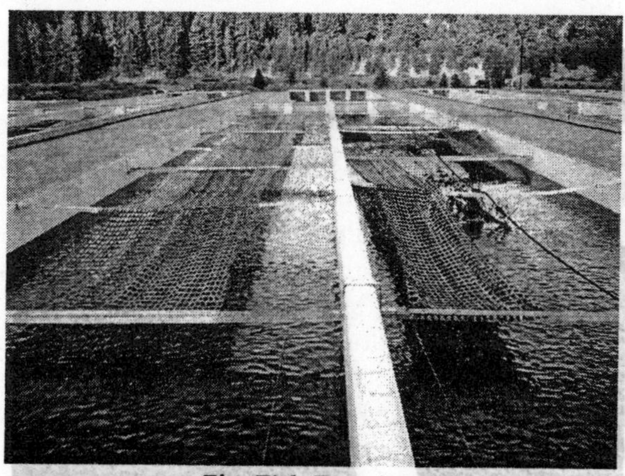

Fig. Fish Farming

Increasing demands on wild fisheries by commercial fishing operations have caused widespread overfishing. Fish farming offers an alternative solution to the increasing market demand for fish and fish protein.

MAJOR CATEGORIES OF FISH FARMS

There are two kinds of aquaculture: extensive aquaculture based on local photosynthetical production and intensive aquaculture, in which the fish are fed with external food supply. The management of these two kinds of aquaculture systems are completely different.

Extensive (pond) Aquaculture

Limiting for fish growth here is the available food supply by natural sources, commonly zooplankton feeding on pelagic algae or benthic animals, such as certain crustaceans and mollusks. Tilapia species filter feed directly on phytoplankton, which makes higher production possible.

The photosynthetical production can be increased by fertilizing the pond water with artificial fertilizer mixtures, such as potash, phosphorus, nitrogen and microelements. Because most fish are carnivorous, they occupy a higher place in the trophic chain and therefore only a tiny fraction of primary photosynthetic production will be converted into harvestable fish.

As a result, without additional feeding the fish harvest will not exceed 200 kilograms of fish per hectare per year, equivalent to 1 per cent of the gross photosynthetic production.

A second point of concern is the risk of algal blooms. When temperatures, nutrient supply and available sunlight are optimal for algal growth, algae multiply their biomass at an exponential rate, eventually leading to an exhaustion of available nutrients and a subsequent die-off. The decaying algal biomass will deplete the oxygen in the pond water because it blocks out the sun and pollute it with organic and inorganic solvents (such as ammonium ions), which can (and frequently do) lead to massive loss of fish.

In order to tap all available food sources in the pond, the aquaculturist will choose fish species which occupy different places in the pond ecosystem, e.g., a filter algae feeder such as tilapia, a benthic feeder such as carp or catfish and a zooplankton feeder (various carps) or submerged weeds feeder such as grass carp.

Intensive (closed-circulation) Aquaculture

In these kinds of systems fish production per unit of

surface can be increased at will, as long as sufficient oxygen, fresh water and food are provided. Because of the requirement of sufficient fresh water, a massive water purification system must be integrated in the fish farm. A clever way to achieve this is the combination of hydroponic horticulture and water treatment. The exception to this rule is cages which are placed in a river or sea, which supplements the fish crop with sufficient fresh water. Environmentalists object to this practice.

The cost of inputs per unit of fish weight is higher than in extensive farming, especially because of the high cost of fish food, which must contain a much higher level of protein (up to 60 per cent) than, e.g., cattle food and a balanced amino acid composition as well. This frequently is offset by the lower land costs and the higher productions which can be obtained due to the high level of input control.

Essential here is aeration of the water, as fish need a sufficient oxygen level for growth. This is achieved by bubbling, cascade flow or aqueous oxygen. Catfish, Clarias ssp. can breathe atmospheric air and can tolerate much higher levels of pollutants than, e.g., trout or salmon, which makes aeration and water purification less necessary and makes *Clarias* species especially suited for intensive fish production. In some *Clarias* farms about 10 per cent of the water volume can consist of fish biomass.

Especially when fish densities are high, the risk of infections by parasites like fish lice, fungi (Saprolegnia ssp.), intestinal worms (such as nematodes or trematodes), bacteria (e.g., Yersinia ssp, Pseudomonas ssp.), and protozoa (such as Dinoflagellates) is much higher than in animal husbandry because of the ease in which pathogens can invade the fish body (e.g. by the gills).

The same holds for water pollution or depletion of oxygen in the water, which can ruin a fish crop within minutes. This means, intensive aquaculture requires tight monitoring and a high level of expertise of the fish farmer.

Intensive aquaculture was developed as a source for food fish. Raising ornamental cold water fish (goldfish or koi), although theoretically much more profitable due to the higher income per weight of fish produced, has never been successfully carried out until very recently.

The increased incidences of dangerous viral diseases of koi Carp, together with the high value of the fish has led to initiatives in closed system koi breeding and growing in a number of countries. Today there are a few commercially successful intensive koi growing facilities in the UK, Germany and Israel.

Some producers have adapted their intensive systems and attempted to make them biosecure in an effort to provide consumers with fish that do not carry dormant forms of viruses and diseases.

SPECIFIC TYPES OF FISH FARMS

Within intensive and extensive aquaculture methods there are numerous specific types of fish farms, each has benefits and applications unique to its design.

Integrated Recycling Systems

One of the largest problems with freshwater aquaculture is that it can use a million gallons of water per acre (about 1 m^3 of water per m^2) each year. Extended water purification systems allow for the reuse (recycling) of local water.

The largest-scale pure fish farms use a system derived (admittedly much refined) from the New Alchemists in the 1970s. Basically, large plastic fish tanks are placed in a greenhouse. A hydroponic bed is placed near, above or between them. When tilapia are raised in the tanks, they are able to eat algae, which naturally grows in the tanks when the tanks are properly fertilized.

The tank water is slowly circulated to the hydroponic beds where the tilapia waste feeds a commercial plant crops. Carefully cultured microorganisms in the hydroponic bed convert ammonia to nitrates, and the plants are fertilized by the nitrates and phosphates. Other wastes are strained out by the hydroponic media, which doubles as an aerated pebble-bed filter.

This system, properly tuned, produces more edible

protein per unit area than any other. A wide variety of plants can grow well in the hydroponic beds. Most growers concentrate on herbs (e.g. parsley and basil), which command premium prices in small quantities all year long. The most common customers are restaurant wholesalers.

Since the system lives in a greenhouse, it adapts to almost all temperate climates, and may also adapt to tropical climates.

The main environmental impact is discharge of water that must be salted to maintain the fishes' electrolyte balance. Current growers use a variety of proprietary tricks to keep fish healthy, reducing their expenses for salt and waste water discharge permits. Some veterinary authorities speculate that ultraviolet ozone disinfectant systems (widely used for ornamental fish) may play a prominent part in keeping the Tilapia healthy with recirculated water. A number of large, well-capitalized ventures in this area have failed. Managing both the biology and markets is complicated.

Irrigation Ditch or Pond Systems

These use irrigation ditches or farm ponds to raise fish. The basic requirement is to have a ditch or pond that retains water, possibly with an above-ground irrigation system (many irrigation systems use buried pipes with headers. Using this method, one can store one's water allotment in ponds or ditches, usually lined with bentonite clay.

In small systems the fish are often fed commercial fish food, and their waste products can help fertilize the fields. In larger ponds, the pond grows water plants and algae as fish food. Some of the most successful ponds grow introduced strains of plants, as well as introduced strains of fish.

Control of water quality is crucial. Fertilizing, clarifying and pH control of the water can increase yields substantially, as long as eutrophication is prevented and oxygen levels stay high.Yields can be low if the fish grow ill from electrolyte stress.

Cage System

Fish cages are placed in open water resources to contain

and protect fish until they can be harvested. They can be constructed of a wide variety of components. Fishes are stocked in cages, artificially fed, and harvested when they reach market size.

A few advantages of fish farming with cages are that many types of waters can be used (rivers, lakes, filled quarries, etc.), many types of fishes can be raised, and fish farming can co-exist with sport fishing and other water uses. Cage farming of fishes in open seas are also gaining popularity. Concerns of disease, poaching, poor water quality, etc., lead some to believe that in general, pond systems are easier to manage and simpler to start. Also, past occurrances of cage-failures leading to escapes, have raised concern regarding the culture of non-native fish species in open-water cages. Even though the cage-industry has made numerous technological advances in cage construction in recent years, the concern for escapes remains valid.

Classic Fry Farming

Trout and other sport fish are often raised from eggs to fry or fingerlings and then trucked to streams and released. Normally, the fry are raised in long, shallow concrete tanks, fed with fresh stream water. The fry receive commercial fish food in pellets.

While not as efficient as the New Alchemists' method, it is also far simpler, and has been used for many years to stock streams with sport fish. European eel (Anguilla anguilla) aquaculturalists procure a limited supply of glass eels, juvenile stages of the European eel which swim north from the Sargasso Sea breeding grounds, for their farms.

The European eel is threatened with extinction because of the excessive catch of glass eels by Spanish fishermen and overfishing of adult eels in, e.g., the Dutch IJsselmeer, Netherlands. As per 2005, no one has managed to breed the European eel in captivity.

ENVIRONMENTALLY FRIENDLY METHODS

An alternative to open ocean cage aquaculture, one in

which the risk of environmental damage is substantially eliminated is through the use of a recirculating aquaculture system (RAS). A RAS is a series of culture tanks and filters where water is continuously recycled. To prevent the deterioration of water quality, the water is treated mechanically through the removal of particulate matter and biologically through the conversion of harmful accumulated chemicals into nontoxic ones.

Other treatments such as UV sterilization, ozonation, and oxygen injection are also utilized to maintain optimal water quality.

Through this system, many of the environmental drawbacks of aquaculture are minimized including escaped fish, water usage, and the introduction of harmful pollutants. The practices also increase efficiency of feed utilisation and growth by providing optimal water quality parameters.

One of the drawbacks to recirculating aquaculture systems is water exchange. However, the rate of water exchange can be reduced through aquaponics, such as the incorporation of hydroponically grown plants and denitrification. Both methods reduce the amount of nitrate in the water, and can potentially eliminate the need for water exchanges, closing the aquaculture system from the environment.

The amount of interaction between the aquaculture system and the environment can be measured through the cumulative feed burden (CFB kg/M^3), which measures the amount of feed that goes into the RAS relative to the amount of water and waste discharged.

Because of its high capital and operating costs, RAS has generally been restricted to practices such as broodstock maturation, larval rearing, fingerling production, research animal production, SPF (specific pathogen free) animal production, and caviar and ornamental fish production. Although the use of RAS for other species is considered by many aquaculturalists to be impractical, there has been some limited successful implementation of this with high value product such as barramundi, sturgeon and live tilapia in the US.

AQUACULTURE FISH

Aquaculture is the cultivation of aquatic organisms. Unlike fishing, aquaculture, also known as aquafarming, implies the cultivation of aquatic populations under controlled conditions. Mariculture refers to aquaculture practiced in marine environments. Particular kinds of aquaculture include algaculture (the production of kelp/seaweed and other algae); fish farming; shrimp farming, shellfish farming, and the growing of cultured pearls.

Aquaculture has been used in China since circa 2500 BC. When the waters lowered after river floods, some fishes, namely carp, were held in artificial lakes. Their brood was later fed using nymphs and silkworm feces, while the fish themselves were eaten as a source of protein. By a fortunate genetic mutation, this early domestication of carp lead to the development of goldfish in the Tang Dynasty.

The Hawaiian people practiced aquaculture by constructing fish ponds. A remarkable example from ancient Hawaii is the construction of a fish pond, dating from at least 1,000 years ago, at Alekoko. According to legend, it was constructed by the mythical Menehune. The Japanese practiced cultivation of seaweed by providing bamboo poles and, later, nets and oyster shells to serve as anchoring surfaces for spores. The Romans often bred fish in ponds.

The practice of aquaculture gained prevalence in Europe during the middle Ages, since fish were scarce and thus expensive. However, improvements in transportation during the 19th century made fish easily available and inexpensive, even in inland areas, causing a decline in the practice.

The first North American fish hatchery was constructed on Dildo Island, Newfoundland Canada in 1889, it was the largest and most advanced in the world. Americans were rarely involved in aquaculture until the late 20th century, but California residents harvested wild kelp and made legal efforts to manage the supply starting circa 1900, later even producing it as a wartime resource.

In contrast to agriculture, the rise of aquaculture is a contemporary phenomenon. About 430 (97 per cent) of the aquatic species presently in culture have been domesticated since the start of the 20th century, and an estimated 106 aquatic species have been domesticated over the past decade. The domestication of an aquatic species typically involves about a decade of scientific research.

Current success in the domestication of aquatic species results from the 20th century rise of knowledge on the basic biology of aquatic species and the lessons learned from past success and failure.

The stagnation in the world's fisheries and overexploitation of 20 to 30 per cent of marine fish species have provided additional impetus to domesticate marine species, just as overexploitation of land animals provided the impetus for the early domestication of land species

In the 1960s, the price of fish began to climb, as wild fish capture rates peaked and the human population continued to rise. Today, commercial aquaculture exists on an unprecedented, huge scale.

In the 1980s, open-netcage salmon farming also expanded; this particular type of aquaculture technology remains a minor part of the production of farmed finfish worldwide, but possible negative impacts on wild stocks, which have come into question since the late 1990s, have caused it to become a major cause of controversy.

TYPES OF AQUACULTURE

Algaculture

Algaculture is a form of aquaculture involving the farming of species of algae. The majority of algae that are intentionally cultivated fall into the category of microalgae, also referred to as phytoplankton, microphytes, or planktonic algae.

Macroalgae, commonly know as seaweed, also have many commercial and industrial uses, but due to their size and the specific requirements of the environment in which they need to grow, they do not lend themselves as readily to cultivation on a large scale as microalgae and are most often harvested wild from the ocean.

Fish Farming

Fish farming is the principal form of aquaculture, while other methods may fall under mariculture. It involves raising fish commercially in tanks or enclosures, usually for food. A facility that releases juvenile fish into the wild for recreational fishing or to supplement a species' natural numbers is generally referred to as a fish hatchery.

Fish species raised by fish farms include salmon, catfish, tilapia, cod, carp, trout and others. Increasing demands on wild fisheries by commercial fishing operations have caused widespread overfishing. Fish farming offers an alternative solution to the increasing market demand for fish and fish protein.

Freshwater Prawn Farming

A freshwater prawn farm is an aquaculture business designed to raise and produce freshwater prawn or shrimp for human consumption. Freshwater prawn farming shares many characteristics with and many of the same problems as, marine shrimp farming.

Unique problems are introduced by the developmental life cycle of the main species. The global annual production of freshwater prawns (excluding crayfish and crabs) in 2003 was about 280,000 tons, of which China produced some 180,000 tons, followed by India and Thailand with some 35,000 tons each. Additionally, China produced about 370,000 tons of Chinese river crab.

Integrated Multi-trophic Aquaculture

Integrated Multi-Trophic Aquaculture (IMTA) is a practice in which the by-products (wastes) from one species are recycled to become inputs (fertilizers, food) for another. Fed aquaculture (e.g. fish, shrimp) is combined with inorganic extractive (e.g. seaweed) and organic extractive (e.g. shellfish) aquaculture to create balanced systems for environmental sustainability (biomitigation), economic stability (product diversification and risk reduction) and social acceptability (better management practices).

"Multi-Trophic" refers to the incorporation of species from different trophic or nutritional levels in the same system. This is one potential distinction from the age-old practice of aquatic polyculture, which could simply be the co-culture of different fish species from the same trophic level. In this case, these organisms may all share the same biological and chemical processes, with few synergistic benefits, which could potentially lead to significant shifts in the ecosystem.

Some traditional polyculture systems may, in fact, incorporate a greater diversity of species, occupying several niches, as extensive cultures (low intensity, low management) within the same pond. The "Integrated" in IMTA refers to the more intensive cultivation of the different species in proximity of each other, connected by nutrient and energy transfer through water, but not necessarily right at the same location.

Ideally, the biological and chemical processes in an IMTA system should balance. This is achieved through the appropriate selection and proportions of different species providing different ecosystem functions. The co-cultured species should be more than just biofilters; they should also be harvestable crops of commercial value.

A working IMTA system should result in greater production for the overall system, based on mutual benefits to the co-cultured species and improved ecosystem health, even if the individual production of some of the species is lower compared to what could be reached in monoculture practices over a short term period. Sometimes the more general term "Integrated Aquaculture" is used to describe the integration of monocultures through water transfer between organisms. For all intents and purposes however, the terms "IMTA" and "integrated aquaculture" differ primarily in their degree of descriptiveness.

These terms are sometimes interchanged. Aquaponics, fractionated aquaculture, IAAS (integrated agriculture-aquaculture systems), IPUAS (integrated peri-urban-aquaculture systems), and IFAS (integrated fisheries-aquaculture systems) may also be considered variations of the IMTA concept.

Mariculture

Mariculture is a specialized branch of aquaculture involving the cultivation of marine organisms for food and other products in the open ocean, an enclosed section of the ocean, or in tanks, ponds or raceways which are filled with seawater. An example of the latter is the farming of marine fish, prawns, or oysters in saltwater ponds. Non-food products produced by mariculture include: fish meal, nutrient agar, jewelries (e.g. cultured pearls), and cosmetics.

Shrimp Farming

A shrimp farm is an aquaculture business for the cultivation of marine shrimp for human consumption. Commercial shrimp farming began in the 1970s, and production grew steeply, particularly to match the market demands of the U.S., Japan and Western Europe. The total global production of farmed shrimp reached more than 1.6 million tonnes in 2003, representing a value of nearly 9,000 million U.S. dollars.

About 75 per cent of farmed shrimp is produced in Asia, in particular in China and Thailand. The other 25 per cent is produced mainly in Latin America, where Brazil is the largest producer. The largest exporting nation is Thailand.

Shrimp farming has changed from traditional, small-scale businesses in Southeast Asia into a global industry. Technological advances have led to growing shrimp at ever higher densities, and broodstock is shipped world-wide. Virtually all farmed shrimp are penaeids (i.e., shrimp of the family *Penaeidae*), and just two species of shrimp—the *Penaeus vannamei* (Pacific white shrimp) and the *Penaeus monodon* (giant tiger prawn)—account for roughly 80 per cent of all farmed shrimp.

These industrial monocultures are very susceptible to diseases, which have caused several regional wipe-outs of farm shrimp populations. Increasing ecological problems, repeated disease outbreaks, and pressure and criticism from both NGOs and consumer countries led to changes in the industry in the late 1990s and generally stronger regulation by governments.

In 1999, a programme aimed at developing and promoting more sustainable farming practices was initiated, including governmental bodies, industry representatives, and environmental organizations.

CRAYFISH CULTURE

Among the best known and most highly esteemed crustaceans are the lobsters *(Homarus* spp.), but they are rivalled as a delicacy by their smaller freshwater counterparts, the crayfishes or crawfishes. (Not to be confused with the marine spiny lobsters, family Palinuridae, sometimes marketed as crayfish or crawfish).

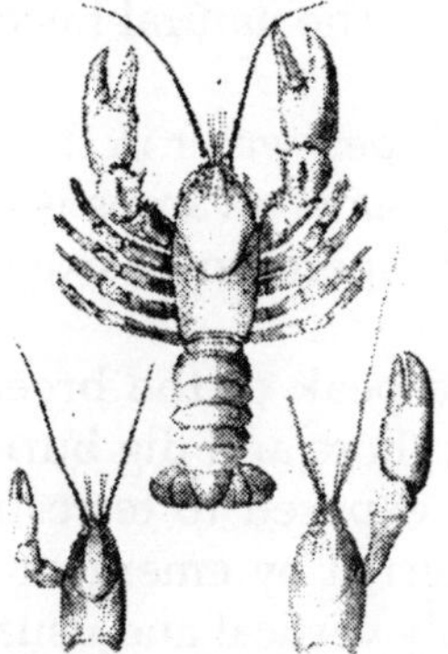

Fig. Cray fish

True crayfish comprise more than 300 species and are found on all the continents except Africa. Although crayfish are esteemed as a gourmet food in several European countries and are the primary source of protein for certain tribes in New Guinea, they are generally underutilized by man.

Crayfish have attained importance as a commercial food product in parts of Europe and the United States. These most enthusiastic consumers of crayfish are the French, and crayfish farms have been in operation in France since 1880. But the most important crayfish producing area is Louisiana, the only American state with a history of French culture. In a good year more than 800,000 kg of "wild" crayfish may be caught and marketed in Louisiana; during bad years the yield may be less than half that figure.

Fishery production is supplemented annually by 1.2 million kg produced on the 6000 to 7000 ha. of crayfish, farms in the state. Details are not available on techniques of crayfish culture in Europe; hence this report concentrates on practices in Louisiana.

NATURAL HISTORY OF THE PRINCIPAL CULTURED SPECIES

There are twenty-nine species of crayfish known to inhabit the waters of Louisiana, but only two are cultured. On most farms the dominant species is the red crayfish *(Procambarus clarkii)*, but a few areas produce chiefly white crayfish *(Procambarus blandingi)*. The natural history of the two species is similar.

Mating occurs in open water in the late spring, when the water level in the Louisiana swamps is high. At that time the male crayfish deposits sperm in an external receptacle on the female.

Shortly after the peak of the breeding season, female crayfish come out on shore and dig burrows near the water's edge. Since they are exposed to terrestrial predators at this time, areas well protected by emergent plants are preferred. Burrows are essentially vertical and usually 0.7 to 1.0 m deep, unless the water table is unusually high, in which case burrows half that depth may be found.

By the end of July, all adult females have constructed burrows, which are then usually occupied by a single male, along with the female. Each burrow is capped with a plug of dirt. Young crayfish and unpaired males also seek shelter in the mud or in naturally occurring holes during the summer, but they do not burrow. Some additional mating may occur in the burrows, but the crayfish are thought to be essentially inactive until September, when egg laying occurs.

Eggs and sperm are simultaneously released by the female and the fertilized eggs attached to the underside of her tail until hatching, which occurs in 14 to 21 days with red crayfish and 17 to 29 days with white crayfish. The adults die soon after hatching. An average hatch is about 400 red crayfish (maximum 700) and somewhat less for white crayfish. Fertilization and egg laying often occur in the burrow, but growth and survival of the 25-mm, free-swimming young is greatly enhanced if open water is available. In years when the water is low in the fall, hatching may occur in the burrow, in which case the young suffer from overcrowding and lack of food. Or the female may crawl off overland in search of water and die of dehydration or be captured by a predator.

Young crayfish usually seek shelter in dense plant growth near shore, and then move out to deeper water as mature. Both red and white crayfish are annual animals, and maturity may be reached in less than 6 months after hatching.

Crabnasdyfish of all ages are omnivorous but prefer animal matter. Nevertheless, most crayfish, both in nature and in culture, must subsist on a predominantly vegetable diet.

Pond Culture in Louisiana

Crayfish culture is practiced in two types of water rice fields and artificial impoundments. The latter, though its large-scale use dates back little more than 20 years, now accounts for more than 80 per cent of the area devoted to crayfish farming.

Site Selection and Construction

As in most other forms of aquaculture, site selection is crucial in pond culture of crayfish. Due to the shallowness of crayfish ponds, it is essential that the land chosen be relatively flat. When the highest point in the pond bottom is covered by 0.3 m of water, depths of over 1 m should not occur in more than 25 per cent of the remaining area. It is not, however, of any particular value if the pond bottom is level. In fact, small elevations in the bottom have the favourable effect of increasing the area available for burrowing of early breeders.

Densely wooded areas are not favoured, since dense shrubbery and trees along pond banks hinder harvesting, shade out desirable aquatic plants, add leaves and debris which decay and reduce oxygen levels, and may keep temperature in the shallows below optimum.

It was in such environments, however, that pond culture of crayfish had its start in Louisiana and 2400 ha. of densely wooded swampland are still in use in an area just west of the Atchafalaya Basin, where conventional pond construction would be extremely difficult. These leveed swamplands are also heavily used by waterfowl, which are extensively hunted in Louisiana.

Soil quality surely has some effect on crayfish production but, in Louisiana at least, the primary consideration is that the soil hold water.

Water supply is of course important, but crayfish are very tolerant of naturally occurring physical and chemical conditions. Aspects of water quality which are of particular importance to the crayfish farmer are temperature and hardness. Optimum temperatures for red crayfish are thought to be 21 to 29°C, but growth is not drastically reduced until the temperature falls below 13°C.

Above 32°C, red crayfish burrow into the mud and become inactive. White crayfish do better at slightly lower temperatures and begin to burrow at temperature as low as 27°C. Growth is the primary reason for the culturist to be concerned with water temperature, since neither species is likely to suffer significant thermally induced mortality at temperatures common in Louisiana. For the same reason, dissolved oxygen concentration, though unlikely to be a cause of mortality, should be kept as high as possible.

Cultured crayfish have been observed to do well at pH levels as low as 5.8 and as high as 8.2. Crayfish in acid waters tend to have thinner shells. Soft water also results in thin, soft shells as well as poor growth and survival. It appears that the water in crayfish ponds should have a total hardness of at least 50 ppm, and that up to 200 ppm is desirable.

In recent years interest in crayfish farming in the coastal swamps of southern Louisiana has increased, and some attention has been paid to the effect of salinity on crayfish. Preliminary experiments indicate that crayfish will reproduce and grow fairly well at salinities of 6 to 10 per cent.

Tolerant as crayfish are to natural conditions, they are

extremely sensitive to synthetic chemicals and other substances which may find their way into agricultural water supplies. Such commonly used compounds as Pyrethrum, creosote, orthodichlorobenzene, sodium cyanide, turpentine, orthocresole, cresylic acid, pine oil, nicotine, carbon bisulfide, phenothiazine, calcium cyanamid, and chlorinated hydrocarbon pesticides have all been shown to be toxic to crayfish.

The last-named group presents particular problems because of the possible danger to human health from dosages sublethal for crayfish and because the crayfish farmer may find it difficult to prevent contamination of his water supply by pesticides used on nearby agricultural land. It is recommended that crayfish culturists located in the vicinity of intensive terrestrial farming operations alert neighbouring farmers and crop-dusting pilots of the location of their crayfish ponds and attempt to secure their cooperation in averting contamination. When spraying is going on nearby, pumping of water from streams and ditches into crayfish ponds should be suspended.

The danger of contamination by pesticides and other pollutants is greatly reduced if the water source is a deep well, but many farmers, for reasons of necessity or economy, use surface water. Whichever type of water is used, it is best if each unit of the farm is provided with its own pump. Units need not be discrete but may be portions of larger ponds separated by inside levees.

The smaller the units, the greater the ease of water quality control and general management. On the other hand, the more small units are built, the greater the construction cost per hectare of water surface. A large farm might consist of one or two 100-to 300-ha ponds broken up into 10 or so units. One-family farms as small as 8 ha exist but do not provide a full family income.

Detailed advice on levee construction may be obtained from the Soil Conservation Service, county agricultural agents, or commercial contractors. In general, levees should be high enough to keep out flood waters and wide enough to permit access to vehicles.

Water circulation has been found to be a deciding factor in the success or failure of many crayfish farms. To facilitate circulation it is necessary to provide not only an adequate inflow of water but good drainage as well. Drain pipes, which must be screened with 12-mm or smaller wire mesh, should be located as far away from pipes as possible to permit thorough mixing of water. Drains should be large enough to permit complete draining in 30 days.

Stocking

Although some ponds contain natural populations of crayfish, stocking is nevertheless necessary the first year, after which the population should be self-sustaining. The usual procedure is to stock ponds with adults in May to July, at which time crayfish are "tough" and prices low.

The pond should be flooded for at least 2 weeks before stocking and arrangements made to purchase freshly caught crayfish. Stock held in captivity for even so short a period as overnight should not be accepted. Large specimens, about 30 to 45/kg. are preferable.

Suggested stocking rates for red crayfish vary according to the amount of cover in the pond. At least 80 per cent of most lots of crayfish purchased for stocking in most parts of Louisiana will be red crayfish.

If as occasionally happens, a stock of predominantly white crayfish is obtained. Crayfish of either species should be placed in the pond as soon as possible and kept cool and damp until that time. Predation on newly stocked crayfish will be reduced if they are released in densely vegetated areas or, if the pond is sparsely vegetated, in deep water far from shore.

The most important management techniques in crayfish culture involve manipulation of water level and quality. Each year ponds are drained in late June or early July, when the females have started burrowing. Slow draining is preferable, for fast draining will strand some crayfish which are not ready to burrow and expose them to predators. Similarly, slow draining allows young crayfish to seek hiding places for the summer.

Ponds are reflooded in September to ensure that the newly hatched young will have ample water. If growth rates are normal, they should be ready for harvest starting in late November or early December. The culturist should keep on an eye rainfall, which is the principal controlling factor on wild crayfish harvests, and time reflooding so that he can begin harvesting before the wild crop comes in. Early crayfish bring the best prices and may spell the difference between economic success and failure.

Ordinarily, harvesting lasts until the pond is drained the following summer. Between reflooding and the onset of the harvest season in ponds having heavy cover, water levels 50 cm or so lower than those recommended above can be maintained to furnish more shallow water for young crayfish.

During the harvesting season the water level should be kept fairly stable. This requires frequent pumping to replace water lost by evaporation. Pumping must also be resorted to replace deoxygenated water. Any abrupt reduction in harvest is usually a sign of deoxygenation or some such condition and calls for partial replacement of water.

Good Supply

Any animal food that cultured crayfish get is the result of natural production and their own foraging, but successful culturists encourage suitable food plants and discourage large, tough plants which interfere with harvesting, shade out smaller, more desirable plants, and are inedible by crayfish. Crayfish from ponds that do not contain adequate amounts of edible plants often have brown or black "fat" or livers, and tails which are not filled out, and are considered to be of inferior quality to well nourished crayfish with full tails and yellow livers.

Plants used as food and/ or cover in crayfish ponds must be capable of survival both while the pond is flooded and when it is dry. The most desired food and cover plant in crayfish ponds is alligator grass *(Alternanthera phylloxeroides).* It can be seeded into a pond by raking it out of ditches and scattering it in the pond during drawdown in June and July.

Alligator grass may, on occasion, grow too thick and hinder harvesting. If harvesting is done by boat, boat trails may be disked or raked on the bottom during the summer. Although cattle should generally be kept out of crayfish culture areas, grazing them on the dry pond bottom may help retard alligator grass.

Water primrose (*Jussiaea* spp.) is now considered as good as or better than alligator grass and may be planted together with it. Water primrose has the advantages of not growing as thick as alligator grass and being more tolerant of cold weather. A number of other plants which occur naturally in crayfish ponds, including pondweeds (*Potamogeton* spp.), *Elodea,* and duckweed (*Lemna),* are fair food and/or cover plants and should not ordinarily be discouraged. It is certain that fertilization of dry ponds would benefit all of these and other plants, but techniques to encourage desired species have yet to be worked out.

Crayfish will also eat almost any soft terrestrial plant. Some farmers have planted sorghum or millet as feed for crayfish and claim increased yields.

It is likely that supplemental feeding with animal matter would increase production, but it is doubtful whether it would be economically feasible. Experiments with feeding young red crayfish at Auburn University showed that growth was better on a diet of *Elodea* and ground *Tilapia* than on either component alone. Research is currently being carried out at Louisiana State University with the aim of developing an economical, high-protein artificial feed for crayfish.

Problems

The most common pest plants in crayfish ponds are cattails (*Typha* spp.) They can usually be controlled only if caught early, at which time individual plants can be pulled out manually. If dense growths occur, disking and raking the pond immediately on drying may be helpful. Otherwise, it is necessary to call on state or federal agencies for assistance.

Outside help is also usually necessary to control water hyacinth (*Eichornia crassipes)* which, unchecked, may completely cover the surface of a pond. A number of emergent plants other than cattails are usually present but seldom reach problematical densities in ponds which are drained and dried annually.

Filamentous green algae, which occur principally during the winter, also may hinder harvesting operations. They are prone to die off suddenly in warm weather, creating a pollution problem. Partial removal of floating algal mats may be effected by vigourous circulation of the water.

Man is by no means the only animal which is fond is crayfish, and predation by fish, birds, raccoons, bullfrogs, snakes, turtles, salamanders, large water beetles, and others, is a problem confronting every crayfish culturist. The best protection against most of these predators is abundant cover in the pond, but fish, the most serious predators, may require additional measures.

Annual draining and drying of course substantially reduce fish populations, but some of the worst predators, notably green sunfish *(Lepomis cyanellus)*, bowfin *(Amia calva)*, and bullheads *(lctalurus* spp.), may survive in potholes until reflooding time. Rotenone at 2 to 3 ppm will destroy such fish. Great care should be exercised in its use, however, and a biologist consulted if possible, since 5 ppm of rotenone will kill some young crayfish.

It is standard practice to screen pond outlets to prevent fish from entering, but opinions differ as to the feasibility of screening inflow pipes. Many successful operators reason that most large fish are killed by the pump impellers and do not screen inflow pipes. In any event, the large 0.3-to 0.7-m pumps employed on most ponds move great volumes of water and make screening difficult.

It is recommended that, on new ponds supplied by surface waters, a temporary screen be installed on the inflow pipe and checked frequently during the first few days. If considerable numbers of large predatory fish are captured, a permanent screen should be employed. A suitable design consists of a cylinder of 25-cm weldwire about 1 m in diameter and 4 m long. Such a screen will allow young of predatory fish to enter the pond, but finer screens clog up very rapidly and require constant cleaning.

Harvesting

The most frequently used harvesting device is an 0.8 to 1.0 m long funnel shaped trap made of 21-cm mesh chicken wire and so constructed that it folds flat for hauling. Shorter traps are fully as effective for capturing crayfish, but dissolved oxygen concentrations may become very low in crowded, submerged traps, causing mortality. Long traps, however, may be propped up at an angle so that a small portion is above the surface of the water, and trapped crayfish can obtain air. Traps are commonly baited with fish heads or chunks of gizzard shad *(Dorosoma cepedianum)*, which, is considered more effective than any other fish. Fresh fish may be scarce during the winter, and soybean cake, perforated cans of dog food, or almost any high-protein substance may be substituted. About 25 traps/ha are set out.

Most of the harvesting is done by professional fishermen hired by the culturist. This compounds the culturist's harvesting problems, since he is seldom able to maintain a crew of fishermen throughout a harvest season. But to realise maximum yields and fulfil contracts to buyers it is essential that harvesting be intensive throughout the season.

The problem is particularly acute during cold weather, when fishermen may be reluctant to run their traps frequently, and during the height of the wild crayfish season, when they may be able to make more money harvesting wild stocks on their own. The demand for labour is particularly great at the start of the season, in late November and early December, when many culturists prefer to harvest as heavily as possible to beat the peak of the wild crop, to utilize adults which have spawned and will die shortly and reduce the danger of crowding of the young crayfish. Crayfish have long been harvested as an incidental crop from rice fields in Louisiana, but it is only in the last 15 years that intensive cultivation has become common. Today, nearly 1000 ha. of rice fields are operated in 2-year rotation as crayfish ponds and pastures.

The approximate schedule for this sort of rotation is given. There are usually enough crayfish present in a Louisiana rice field to serve as brood stock. If not, adults may be stocked at 6 to 12 kg/ha during May. Some crayfish leave the drained fields in July and August, but most of them burrow into the moist soil.

Rice stubble resprouts about a week after harvest, at which time the fields are reflooded to a depth of 15 to 45 cm. Crayfish in rice fields feed mainly on rice stubble and various aquatic plants which find their way into the fields. Rice-crayfish farmers should not use rice seed treated with aldrin, which may be toxic to crayfish.

Harvesting crayfish from rice fields, although tedious, is easier and cheaper than in ponds. Due to the more regular bottom, nets may be employed. The usual type, called a drop net or umbrella net, consists of a rectangular piece of netting, each corner of which is connected by a wire or rod to a ring located over the centre of the net.

A pole or other lifting device is inserted in this ring and the net laid flat on the bottom. Crayfish are baited into it with beef pancreas or other offal and captured by lifting the pole. Ordinary farm labourers rather than professional fishermen may be hired to do this chore.

Growth to the minimum marketable size of 10 to 15 9 is rapid in either type of culture, requiring little more than 6 months. Larger 40-to 45-g crayfish, which bring the best prices, are harvested principally in the early part of the season and may be 8 to 14 months old. Well-managed ponds and rice fields commonly produce 400 to 700 kg/ha of crayfish, and yields of better than 1100 kg/ha have been achieved.

Marketing is by no means organized. Crayfish may be sold live, boiled; or as peeled tails to wholesale dealers, restaurants, or individuals. Production or peeled tails may be increased if a mechanical crayfish peeler, currently being developed at Louisiana State University, is perfected.

INDIAN CARPS

It has become a cliche that the people of India need

protein. Even the most socially unaware persons have some grasp of the magnitude of India's problem. One can cite statistics *ad infinitum* to demonstrate that India is in a steadily worsening state of nutritional crisis, but however one defines the problem, it is clear that the solution, if there is ever to be one, will not come as any single panacea, but from effective population control coupled with increased and more efficient protein production by many means, including fish culture.

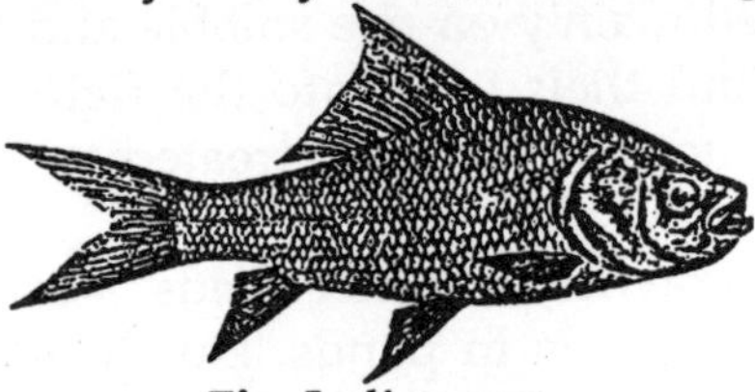

Fig. Indian crap

Fish culture shows promise in India, for there is a considerable demand for fish (total landings of fish in 2003 amounted to 7331 thousand metric tons), a number of native fish well suited to culture; a tradition of fish culture, and a great abundance of cultivable waters (an estimated 7,307,642 ha of fresh and brackish water).

As elsewhere in Asia, the most commonly cultured fish in India and Pakistan are members of the carp family (Cyprinidae). Indian cyprinids used in fish culture are popularly separated into two groups the most desirable species are referred to as major carps; the smallest less desirable species are called minor carps.

The minor carps persist in Indian fish culture largely because as fry they are extremely difficult to distinguish from the major carps, and are thus unintentionally stocked. Minor carps may also be deliberately stocked when stocks of major carps are scarce. In the south of India, in the states of Madras and Mysore, a third group, the Cauvery carps, largely supplant the major carps.

Indian carps have not yet become as popular for introduction and culture outside their native habitat as the common carp *(Cyprinus carpio)* or the Chinese carps, but the catla *(Catla catla)* has been introduced to Ceylon, experimentally cultured in Israel and the United States, and commercially raised in Malaysia. All the Indian major carps have been recommended for use in the Philippines.

The major carps comprise the catla, the rohu *(Labeo rohita)*, and the mrigal *(Cirrhinus mrigala)*. Some authorities also include the calbasu *(Labeo calbasu)*. These three or four species are often grown in polyculture, though their ecological niches are by no means as distinct and well defined as those of the Chinese carps, nor is Indian polyculture nearly as sophisticated as the ancient Chinese practice.

In general, the catla feeds on plankton and decayed macro vegetation on the surface and throughout the water column, the rohu is a column feeder on decayed vegetation with a taste for higher plants, the mrigal a bottom-feeding herbivore, and the calbasu a benthic omnivore. Certain of the Chinese carps have been experimentally included in Indian carp polyculture systems and in the future further combinations of Indian carps, Chinese carps, and other fish may be expected in both experimental and practical culture.

The niches of the Cauvery carps overlap; thus polyculture of these three species could probably be enhanced by introduction of other species. The species association for fish culture in southern India has already been diversified by the introduction of catla. The catla joins the fringe-lipped carp *(Labeo fimbriatus)*, which consumes mostly filamentous algae and some zooplankton; the white carp *(Cirrhinus cirrhosa)*, a plankton feeder with a preference for zooplankton, and the Cauvery carp *(Labeo kontius)*, which competes with the fringe-lipped carp for filamentous algae, but also eats pieces of plants and detritus.

Minor carps present in fish ponds vary from region to region. Among those commonly found in one or another part of India are the reba *(Cirrhinus reba)*, which feeds largely on phytoplankton and decayed plants; the nagendram fish *(Osteochilus thomassi)*, a benthic and marginal feeder on filamentous algae and diatoms; and the sandkhol carp *(Thynnichthys sandkhol)*, which consumes mostly phytoplankton plus some zooplankton; also the bata *(Labeo bata)*, the carnatic carp *(Barbus carnaticus), Barbus chola, Labeo boga, Labeo dyoechilus, Labeo gonius, Labeo nandina,* and *Barbus sarana.*

One more Indian cyprinid should be mentioned: the omnivorous copper mahseer *(Barbus hexagonolepis).* Not exactly a "minor" carp, the copper mahseer attains a maximum length of 90 cm. It is cultured in some parts of India but is not included in the traditional Indian polycultural scheme.

For many years a major obstacle to the development of culture of the Indian carps has been the inability of culturists to consistently breed them in captivity. All species spawn naturally in rivers and will not reproduce in standing water, although the major carps may be spawned in specially constructed reservoirs, or bunds, where there is enough current to approximate river conditions.

The copper mahseer will also spawn in running water ponds provided the temperature is about 20°C, or ripe fish may be hand stripped and the eggs fertilized artificially. Little or no effort has been expended on hand stripping or reservoir spawning of the Cauvery carps or minor carps.

The technique of bund spawning can be applied only where the drainage from an extensive catchment area can be accumulated in a natural depression. The low end of such a depression is blocked off by a strong embankment, so that during the rainy season intermittent streams will inundate the depression. Or a dam may be built in the uplands to concentrate runoff in one place, from which it is channelled into the bund.

During the dry season a minimum of 1.5 m of water is maintained in a pool perhaps 3000 m^2 in area, which is stocked with catla, rohu, mrigal, and calbasu in a 4: 2: 1: 1 ratio at a sex ratio of 2 males per female; males may be distinguished by the rough dorsal surface of the pectoral fin. The exact number of fish stocked depends on the extent of the spawning area; about 1 fish per 15 m^2 is appropriate. The pool is usually fished just before the start of the monsoon, and the numbers of each species and sex estimated, so that losses can be rectified by stocking.

The spawning area is a flat piece of land on which grass

is grown during the dry season so that the water will not be easily muddied when it is flooded. It may comprise the entire bund other than the permanent pool, or it may be just one corner of the bund. When the rains come and flood the spawning ground an outlet channel in the embankment is opened up so that water circulates through the bund. The breeders then move out of the pool and begin chasing in the shallow areas. Spawning usually occurs at night during the full moon or new moon. When spawning is completed, the eggs are collected by dragging seines, about 4 m long x 1.5 m deep, made of mosquito netting, over the spawning ground. Unfortunately a large percentage of the eggs is often destroyed by being trampled by the fishermen.

The eggs are placed in spawning pits dug as near as possible to the bund and supplied with bund water. These pits may be 1 to 1.3 m long, 0.6 m wide and 0.3 m deep and accommodate from 100,000 to 300,000 eggs. When the inlet to the pit is closed, the water temperature rises rapidly, accelerating hatching time to 12 to 18 hours, instead of the 36 hours that might be required at lower temperatures.

The rate of hatching in these pits is low due to bacterial decay and lack of aeration in the stagnant water. Some improvement may be effected by suspending a hatching net or "hapa" in a hatching pit. The hapa is rectangular in shape and constructed as a net within a net. The eggs are placed in the inner net, which is made of material just fine enough to hold them. The newly hatched larvae pass through into the outer net of fine cloth and are nursed there until they are 4 to 5 days old, by which time they have become fry.

The technique of bund spawning may be used only in areas where the topography permits. Induced spawning with the aid of pituitary injections is more generally applicable. The first attempts to apply this technique to the Indian carps were made in 1956, but it is only in the last five or six years that consistent success has been achieved. Today all four major carps and a number of other Indian cyprinids are bred in this manner. Success has been found to hinge on the quality of pituitary glands used and the correct dosage.

Pituitaries used in induction should be taken from fully mature, ripe, or freshly spawned fish of the same species as the fish being spawned, or a very closely related species. Dosage is variable, depending on the stage of maturity of the breeders. Since best results are obtained only with fully mature fish, only dosages for such fish will be described.

Breeders are usually selected from 1.5-to 5.0-kg, 2-to 4 year-old fish stocked in spawning ponds a few months prior to the breeding season, which usually coincides with the southwest monsoon; then segregated at maturity. Maturity of males is easily determined; fully mature specimens ooze milt when the abdomen is gently pressed. Selection of females is more difficult, but fish with soft, rounded, bulging abdomens and swollen, reddish vents are preferred. A catheter may also be used to assess ripeness.

Intramuscular injections are made on the caudal peduncle or near the shoulder region Females are injected two or three times, while males receive only one injection. The first injection, of females only, consists of 2 to 3 mg of pituitary extract/kg of body weight, after which the sexes remain separated for 6 more hours. Then males are given a dose equal to the first injection administered to females, while the females receive a second dose of 5 to 8 mg/kg.

Following this injection, the fish are placed together in groups of three (two males and one female) in covered breeding hapas, 1.6 to 6.5 m2 in surface area and 0.9 m deep fixed on bamboo poles in the marginal waters of ponds. Spawning ordinarily takes place within 3 to 6 hours, but if after 10 to 12 hours no spawning occurs, females only are given a third, slightly higher dosage of pituitary extract.

If the water temperature is near optimum (about 27°C for most species), 60 to 100 per cent success may be expected by this method. Once the eggs have hardened, 8 to 10 hours after spawning, they are transferred, in batches of 75,000 to 1,000,000, to 1.6-m2, 0.9-m deep hatching hapas set in marginal waters of ponds, where they hatch in 15 to 18 hours at 27 to 31°C. Spawners may be sacrificed to obtain their pituitary glands.

As induced spawning of cyprinids becomes more prevalent in India, selective breeding and hybridization of Indian carps can assume greater importance. Experimental hybridization of Indian carps with each other and with Chinese carps has already been done, but the resulting offspring have for the most part been unpromising if not incapable of survival.

One exception is the hybrid catla x -rohu, which combines the wide body of the catla with the small head of the rohu. These traits would give it an advantage at the market wherever consumers do not eat the head of the fish, while at the same time effectively giving the consumer more nourishment for his money. The catla x rohu hybrid is fertile and has produced a healthy F2 generation.

Despite recent improvements in induced spawning methods, the main source of stock for culture in India and Pakistan continues to be collections of eggs, larvae, fry, and fingerlings taken from rivers.

COLLECTION AND HATCHING OF EGGS

Eggs are collected only from the Halda River in the Chittagong area of Bangladesh. Drifting fertilized eggs are captured 12 to 14 hours after spawning, which generally takes place within 3 weeks before or after each full moon from April through July. The precise time of peak spawning is determined by test collections at the start of the season.

The number of eggs caught in these collections enables the collectors to forecast the peak of spawning so that they can fish about that time or shortly after, when the maximum number of eggs is available.

The net used in egg collecting is simple, consisting of no more than a rectangular piece of mosquito netting 11 to 12 m long and 2.7 m wide with a bamboo pole attached at each end. Such nets are usually operated by two men in a boat stationed at right angles to the current, but they may also be moored in the river or used by men wading.

Captured eggs may be placed in a compartment of the collecting boat for some time, even up to hatching, but these results in high mortality due to congestion and inadequate aeration. Better methods of holding and hatching eggs involve nets suspended from a bamboo framework, bamboo baskets lined with fine cloth and suspended in the river, or hatching pits dug in the river bank and supplied with water through a system of pipes.

Suspended nets are more often used as a temporary device to accommodate the eggs immediately upon collection, after which the eggs are transferred to pits or baskets, which are believed to produce healthier larvae. A typical hatching pit was 448 cm long x 244 cm wide x 46 cm deep and could accommodate 120 to 300 kg of eggs (900,000 to 2,200,000 eggs).

The hatching rate in all these traditional devices is usually 25 to 50 per cent. Somewhat better results may be obtained using hatching pits in conjunction with the double net device already described in connection with bund spawning.

NURSERY PONDS

Perennial ponds have the serious disadvantage of harbouring a host of predators, parasites, and competitors of carp fry, which seldom can be entirely eliminated. For this reason, in stocking perennial ponds it is best to scatter the fish, rather than dumping them all in at once. Stocking at night is also advisable, since most fry predators feed visually and the fry are especially vulnerable to predation during the period of acclimatization to a new environment. Captured and conditioned fingerlings may be placed directly into growing ponds to fatten them for consumption or stocked in rearing ponds for further intensive care.

Fry, however, must be nursed for 12 to 15 days to insure their health and satisfactory growth. Both seasonal and perennial ponds, ranging from 7 m2 to 0.5 ha in area and 0.9 to 3.6 m deep, are used as nurseries. Sample stocking rates for nursing ponds. Temporary ponds are somewhat better, but the ideal is a pond which can be drained at the discretion of the culturist.

In the relatively few modernized nursery units in India, the ponds are drained and sun-dried before use, the bottom is plowed, and a short-season crop of legu-minous plants is grown as a source of nitrogen for the soil. After harvesting the legume crop, the plants are plowed under and the bottom is leveled.

Fertilization may be carried out using various kinds of manure or refuse, mixed with oil cake, applied at 200 to 325 kg/ha before the pond is filled. Vegetable manures are usually applied in heaps, weighted down with stones rather than scattered about the pond, so as to reduce the danger of widespread deoxygenation.

Animal manure is placed in bags or baskets for the same reason. Dilute sewage is used as a fertilizer in some areas, notably in the Bidyadhuri Spill in Calcutta. In using sewage, care should be taken that the dissolved oxygen concentration in the pond does not drop below 3 ppm. Inorganic fertilizers, though too expensive for use by many culturists, have been used on an experimental basis.

They would appear to be especially promising for use in arid areas, where organic manures are relatively scarce and more appropriately used as a source of humus for the soil. Unfortunately, most of the research on inorganic pond fertilization in India has involved use of the N-P-K mixtures, with little testing of the individual elements.

Use of N-P-K mixtures may be wasteful, as limnological data from many parts of India show an abundance of potassium. The nitrogen-fixing blue-green algae so prevalent in Indian fish ponds, along with the occasional practice of growing legumes in dry ponds, may make the addition of nitrogen superfluous as well.

There is some experimental evidence that phosphates alone are as effective as or better than N-P-K mixtures in many situations, but the lack of adequate controls in this research leaves room for doubt. In parts of Bangladesh a 3: 1 mixture of cow dung and superphosphate is applied to ponds at 555 kg/(ha) (year). Clearly, pond fertilization practices in India and Pakistan can be improved, through research and by greater appreciation of the fact that the waters of the region vary widely in chemical characteristics, so that each body should be treated individually rather than according to some custom or general formula. If the soil is acid, it may also be necessary before filling to treat the pond with lime until a *pH* of 8 or 9 is reached. Large perennial ponds are generally acid, but 300 to 500 kg/ha of lime are usually sufficient to correct this situation.

In ponds which cannot be drained and dried, pest control is a major preoccupation of the culturist. Predators include fish such as the snakeheads *(Ophicephalus* spp.), frogs, and several va-rieties of insect and aquatic birds. Competitors of the carp fry include many species of small, commercially undesirable fish as well as tadpoles. Fishing is usually inadequate to control predator and competitor fish, and poisoning must often be relied on. A number of pesticides of plant origin are used, but the most common is derris root powder. Applied at 4 to 6 ppm, it eliminates virtually all fish as well as killing some aquatic insects and tadpoles.

Larger doses may be more effective, but the prescribed dosage is preferred since it initially only stuns the fish, and edible predators can be salvaged by quickly transferring them to clear water. Control of insects can be achieved by applying an emulsion of 56 kg of mustard or coconut oil and 18 kg of washing soap per hectare. These poisons lose their effectiveness within 2 to 12 days of application, at which time manuring or stocking may be initiated. Ducks and geese must be fenced out of nursery ponds.

Weeds may also cause a problem by competing for nutrients with plankton and by providing hiding places for predators. Manual or mechanical removal is preferable to chemical control, but the possibility of ecological control using shading or herbivorous fishes, should be considered. A lengthier treatment of weed control methods follows in the discussion of growing ponds.

PROBLEMS OF INDIAN CARP CULTURE

Depending on the plant species to be dealt with, a diversity of methods, including poisoning, is used in weed control. Many of the most effective poisons are chlorinated hydrocarbons such as 2,4–, which are scarcely to be recommended for introduction into ecosystems or human food supplies. Other poisons, such as copper sulfate, sodium arsenite, and anhydrous ammonia gas, lack the long-term cumulative effects and the dangers to man presented by the chlorinated hydrocarbons, but they may be toxic to fish. In all but the most desperate cases therefore, it is safer (and usually cheaper) to use mechanical or ecological methods of plant control.

For floating weeds, outright manual removal is the best treatment. Emergent plants may be controlled by cutting of leaves at weekly intervals for about 6 to 8 weeks before fruiting. Marginal weeds may be controlled by many methods, including plowing under, grazing by livestock, burning during the dry season, or deepening the margin of the pond. Rooted sub-merged weeds may be removed, albeit with considerable labour, by netting with strong nets, by dragging chains, or with the aid of various types of fork and rake.

The commonest agents of ecological weed control are herbivorous fish. The most commonly used species for this purpose is the grass carp, which in addition to destroying or reducing most submerged and emergent plants and adding to pond fish production, contributes to the nour-ishment of other fish by dropping partially digested plant remains in its feces. All four of the major carps and a number of the minor carps, although unable to utilize fresh macrophytes as food, consume the partially decayed plant material in grass carp feces. However, grass carp are not a panacea for weed problems, since there are some plants, such as Eichornia and Salvinia, which they eat only with reluctance if at all.

There is also the possibility that if grass carp find their way into natural waterways, they may be destructive of the native flora. Another herbivore, already intro-duced to Ceylon for use in weed control, is the tawes (Barbus gonionotus). A number of species of tilapia, including Tilapia melanopleura, Tilapia mossambica, Tilapia nilotica, and Tilapia zillii, may effectively control certain types of weed. However, T. mossambica has on at least one occasion been found to depress total yield in polyculture involving catla.

Another ecological method of weed control is shading.

Trees around the border of a pond may provide sufficient shade to discourage marginal weeds, but to control offshore weeds in most ponds the culturist must rely either on floating plants such as duckweed (Lemna), individuals of which are small enough not to interfere with netting and routine management operations, or on creation of an algal bloom. A heavy bloom can be induced by repeated application of N-P-K fertilizers, but this may be prohibitively expensive.

An unusual combination of effects results from application of superphosphate or urea at 50 ppm or more. These substances at that concentration are toxic to most submerged plants, but they act as fertilizers and produce an algal bloom as well. The desirability of an algal bloom must of course be evaluated in terms of the characteristics of the individual pond and the feeding habits of the fish present.

Other pond management practices used in India and Pakistan include the treatment of foul water by doses of 1.5 ppm or less of potassium permanganate, raking the pond bottom to release accumulated gases, and addition of minute amounts of alum to settle suspended or colloidal matter and reduce turbidity.

SHEEP FARMING

Domestic sheep are quadrupedal, cloven-hoofed mammals kept as livestock. Though technically the term "sheep" applies to any species in the genus *Ovis*, in everyday use it almost always refers to domestic sheep. Domestic sheep are the most numerous of their genus, and are most likely descended from the wild mouflon. Sheep were one of the earliest animals to be domesticated for agricultural purposes, and are primarily valued for their fleece and meat.

A sheep's wool is the most widely used of any animal, and is typically harvested by shearing. Ovine meat is called lamb when from younger animals and mutton when from older ones. They continue to be important for wool and meat today, and are also occasionally raised for pelts, as dairy animals, or as model organisms for science.

Sheep husbandry is practised throughout the inhabited

world, and has played a pivotal role in many civilizations. In the modern era, Australia, New Zealand, Patagonian nations, and the United Kingdom are most closely associated with sheep production. Sheep-raising has a large lexicon of unique terms which vary considerably by region and dialect.

Use of the word "sheep" began in Middle English as a derivation of the Old English word *scçap*; it is both the singular and plural name for the animal. A group of sheep is called a flock, herd or mob. Adult female sheep are referred to as ewes, intact males as rams, castrated males as wethers, and younger sheep as lambs. Many other specific terms for the various life stages of sheep exist, generally related to lambing, shearing, and age.

Being a key animal in the history of farming, sheep have a deeply entrenched place in human culture, and finds representation in much modern language and symbology. As livestock, sheep are most-often linked to pastoral. Sheep figure in many mythologies—such as the Golden Fleece—and major religions, especially the Abrahamic traditions. In both ancient and modern religious ritual, sheep are used as sacrificial animals. In contemporary English language usage, people who are timid, easily led, or stupid are often compared to sheep.

DESCRIPTION

Domestic sheep are ruminating bovids, typically with horns forming a lateral spiral and crimped hair called wool. Domestic sheep differ from their wild relatives and ancestors in several respects. Wild sheep have uncrimped hair and short tails. Some primitive breeds of domestic sheep have such tails, but a long tail seems to have been an early result of domestication.

Depending on breed, domestic sheep may have no horns at all (polled), or horns in both sexes (as in wild sheep), or in males only. Most horned breeds have a single pair, but some may have several more. Another trait which is unique to *Ovis aries* is its wide variation in colour. Wild sheep breeds are largely variations of solid agouti or brown hues. Colours present in domestic sheep range from pure white to dark chocolate brown and even spotted or piebald. In contemporary culture, the "fluffy white sheep" is an ubiquitous image.

Selection for more easily dyeable white fleeces began early in the history of sheep domestication, and white wool being a dominant trait in sheep it spread quickly. However, coloured sheep do appear in many modern breeds, and may even appear recessively in entirely white flocks. While white fleeces are more sought after for large commercial markets, there is an entrenched niche market for coloured fleeces, mostly for handspinning.

Sheep have a rather wide range of height and weight, largely depending on breed. The rate of a sheep's growth and their eventual mature weight is a highly heritable trait that is often a point of focus for selective breeding. Ewes typically weigh between 100 and 225 pounds (45–100 kg), and rams (being generally larger than ewes) between 100 and 350 pounds (45–160 kg). Mature sheep have 32 teeth.

There are six molars and six premolars, all paired in the upper and lower jaws, together forming broad grinding surfaces at the back of the mouth. The eight incisors (as in other ruminants), are all in the lower jaw, biting against a hard, toothless pad in the upper jaw; together these are used to pick off vegetation. There are no canines, but there is a large gap where they would be, between the incisors and the premolars.

Until the age of four (when all the adult teeth have erupted), it is possible to distinguish the age of sheep from their front teeth: a pair of incisors erupts each year. The front teeth are gradually lost as sheep begin to age, making it progressively harder for them to feed and thus hindering the health and productivity of the animal.

For this reason, domestic sheep on normal pasture begin to decline slowly from four years on, and the average life expectancy of a sheep is 10 to 12 years—though some sheep may live as long as 20 years. Sheep have good hearing, and are sensitive to noise when being handled. Sheep have horizontal slit-shaped pupils, and possess a wide peripheral field of vision with some ability to distinguish colour.

With what is estimated to be approximately 270° to 320°

of wide-angle vision, sheep can see behind themselves without turning their heads (though this ability may be impaired slightly by any wool present around the eyes). However, sheep have poor depth perception; shadows and dips in the ground may cause sheep to balk. In general, sheep have a tendency to want to move out of darkness and in to well-lit areas.

Sheep have an excellent sense of smell, and—like all species of their genus—have scent glands located on their face just in front of the eyes, and interdigitally on the feet. The purpose of these glands is not known for certain, but those on the face are likely to be related to breeding behaviour. The interdigital glands may also be related to sexual selection, but alternative reasons, such as secretion of a waste product or a scent marker to help lost sheep find their flock, have also been posited.

Sheep and goats are closely related (both are in the subfamily Caprinae), and it can sometimes be difficult to differentiate them by appearance alone. However, the genes of sheep and goats differ so greatly that cross-species hybrids rarely occur, and are always infertile. A hybrid of a ewe and a buck (a male goat) is called a sheep-goat hybrid, and is not to be confused with the genetic chimera called a geep.

Visual clues to differentiating sheep and goats include the beard and divided upper lip of goats, which sheep do not have. Sheep tails also hang down, even when short or docked, while the tails of goats are held upwards. Sheep breeds are also often naturally polled (either in both sexes or just in the female), while naturally polled goats are rare (though many are polled artificially). Males of the two species differ especially in that buck goats acquire a unique and very strong odor during the rut, whereas rams do not.

Behaviour

Sheep are prey animals with a strong gregarious instinct, and a majority of sheep behaviours can be defined in these terms. When sheep gather in larger social groups, it provides a mode of defence for a species without another means of doing so. All sheep exhibit some degree of natural flocking behaviour, varying with breed. The dominance hierarchy of wild *Ovis aries* and its natural inclination to follow a leader to new pastures were the pivotal factors in it being one of the first domesticated livestock species. Farmers exploit these behaviours to keep sheep together on open pastures and to move them more easily. Shepherds may also use sheepdogs in this effort, whose highly bred herding ability can assist in moving flocks. In regions such as Iceland, where sheep have no natural predators, none of the native breeds of sheep exhibit a strong flocking behaviour.

Sheep without a flocking instinct tend to scatter rather than stay together when threatened, in a similar manner to goats. It is virtually impossible to use herding dogs with such breeds. Sheep can also become hefted to one particular local pasture (heft) so they do not roam freely in unfenced landscapes. Hefting is an instinct most common in British upland breeds. Ewes teach the heft to their lambs, and if whole flocks are culled it must be retaught to the replacement animals. Flock dynamics in sheep are as a rule only exhibited in a group of four or more sheep.

Fewer sheep may not react as normally expected when alone or with very few other sheep. This is one reason why three is the minimum number of sheep in a sheepdog trial; it places the greatest pressure on a dog's herding abilities. For sheep, the primary defence mechanism is simply to flee from danger when their flight zone is crossed. Secondarily, cornered sheep may attempt to leap at and ram threats in order to escape.

This is particularly true for ewes with newborn lambs and rams (hence the verb form of the word ram). In displaying flocking, sheep have a strong lead-follow tendency, and a leader often as not is simply the first sheep to move. However, sheep do establish a pecking order through physical displays of dominance. Dominant animals are inclined to be more aggressive with other sheep, and usually feed first at troughs. Relationships in flocks tend to be closest among related sheep: in mixed-breed flocks same-breed subgroups tend to form, and a ewe and her direct descendants often move as a unit within very large flocks. Sheep are frequently thought of as extremely stupid animals. A sheep's herd mentality and quickness to flee and panic in the face of stress often make shepherding a difficult endeavor for the uninitiated. Despite these perceptions, a University of Illinois monograph on sheep found them to be just below pigs and on par with cattle in IQ, and some sheep have shown problem-solving abilities; a flock in Yorkshire, England found a way to get over cattle grids by rolling on their backs.

If worked with patiently sheep may learn their names, and many sheep are trained to be led by halter for showing and other purposes. Very rarely, sheep are used as pack animals. Tibetan nomads distribute baggage equally throughout a flock as it is herded between living sites.

Reproduction

Sheep follow a similar reproductive strategy to other herd animals. A flock of ewes is generally mated by a single ram, who has either been chosen by a farmer or has established its dominance through physical contest with other rams (in feral populations). Most sheep are seasonal breeders, though some are able to breed (also called tupping) year-round. Ewes generally reach sexual maturity at six to eight months of age, and rams generally at four to six (ram lambs have occasionally been known to impregnate their mothers at two months).

Ewes enter in to estrus cycles about every 17 days, lasting for approximately 30 hours. In addition to emitting a scent, they indicate their readiness through physical displays towards rams. Sheep may alternatively display a preference for homosexuality, and the behaviour occurs in about eight percent of rams on average. Its occurrence does not seem to be related to flock hierarchy (as some homosexual behaviour is in mammals), rather the ram's typical motor pattern for intercourse is merely directed at rams instead of ewes.

The phenomenon of the freemartin, a female bovine that is behaviourally masculine and lacks functioning ovaries, is most commonly associated with cattle, but does occur to a less extent in sheep. The instance of freemartins in sheep may be increasing in concert with the rise in twinning (freemartins are the result of male-female twin combinations).

Without human intervention, rams fight during the rut to determine which individuals may mate with ewes. Rams, especially unfamiliar ones, will also fight outside the breeding period to establish dominance; rams can kill one another if allowed to mix freely. During the rut, even normally friendly rams may become dangerous to humans due to increased hormone levels.

Historically, especially aggressive rams were sometimes blindfolded or hobbled when interaction with people was necessary. Today, those who keep rams typically prefer softer preventative measures, such as moving within a clear line to an exit, never turning their back on a ram, and possibly using dousing with water or a diluted solution of bleach or vinegar to dissuade charges.

Without ultrasound or other special tools, ascertaining whether sheep are in fact pregnant is initially difficult. Ewes only begin to visibly show a pregnancy about six weeks before the birth, so shepherds sometimes merely rely on the assumption that a ram has been given enough time to impregnate all the ewes. However, a very commonly used piece of equipment for discerning which ewes have been mated with is a marking harness.

By fitting a ram with a chest harness that holds a special crayon (or *raddle*), ewes that have been mounted are marked with its colour. Dye may also be directly applied to the ram's brisket. After mating, sheep have a gestation period of around five months. Within a few days of the impending birth, ewes begin to behave differently.

They may lay down and stand erractically, paw the ground, or otherwise act out of sync with normal flock patterns. A ewe's udder will quickly fill out, and her vulva will swell. Vaginal, uterine or anal prolapse may also occur in problem cases, in which case either stitching or a physical retainer is used to hold the orifice in.

When birth is imminent, contractions begin to take place, and the fitful behaviour of the ewe may increase. A normal labour may take one to several hours: depending on how many lambs are present, the age of the ewe, and her physical and nutritional condition prior to the birth. Though some breeds may regularly throw larger litters of lambs, most produce either single or twin lambs.

At some point, usually either at the beginning of labour or soon after the births have occurred, ewes and lambs may be confined to small lambing jugs. These pens, which are generally two to eight feet in length and width, are designed to facilitate both careful observation of ewes and to cement the bond between them and their lambs.

Ovine obstetrics is sometimes a problematic phenomenon. However, it is a myth that sheep cannot lamb without human assistance: many ewes give birth directly in pasture without aid. While the majority of births are relatively normal and do not require intervention, there are still a number of possible complications that may arise. A lamb may present in the normal fashion (with both legs and head forward), but may simply be too large to slide out of the birth canal.

This often happens when large rams are crossed with diminutive ewes (this is related to breed, rams are naturally larger than ewes by comparison). Lambs may also present themselves with one shoulder to the side, completely backward, or with only some of their limbs protruding. Lambs may also be aborted or stillborn. Some types of abortion in sheep are preventable through a vaccination administered before conception.

In the case of any such problems, those present at lambing (who may or may not include a veterinarian, most shepherds become accomplished at lambing to some degree) may assist the ewe in extracting or repositioning lambs. After the birth, ewes ideally break the amniotic sac (if it is not broken during labour), and begin licking clean the lamb. The licking both clears the nose and mouth, dries the lamb, and stimulates it. Lambs that are breathing and healthy at this point begin trying to stand, and ideally do so between an half and full hour, with help from the mother.

Generally after lambs stand, the umbilical cord is trimmed

to about an inch (2.54 centimeters). Once trimmed, a small container (such as a film canister) of iodine is held against the lamb's belly over the remainder of the cord to prevent infection. In normal situations, lambs nurse after standing, receiving vital colostrum milk. Lambs that either fail to nurse or are prevented from doing so by the ewe require aid in order to live. If coaxing the pair to accept nursing does not work, one of several steps may then be taken. Ewes may be held or tied to force them to accept a nursing lamb. If a lamb is not eating, a stomach tube may also be used to force feed the lamb in order to save its life. In the case of a permanently rejected lamb, a shepherd may then attempt to foster an orphaned lamb onto another ewe.

Lambs are also sometimes fostered after the death of their mother, either from the birth or other event. Scent plays a large factor in ewes recognizing their lambs, so disrupting the scent of a newborn lamb with washing or over-handling may cause a ewe to reject theirs. Conversely, various methods of imparting the scent of a ewe's own lamb to an orphaned one may be useful in fostering. If an orphaned lamb cannot be fostered, then it usually becomes what is known as a bottle lamb—a lamb raised by people and fed via bottle.

After lambs are stabilized, lamb marking—the process of ear tagging, docking, and castrating—is carried out. Vaccinations are usually carried out at this point as well. Ear tags with numbers are the primary mode of identification when sheep are not named; it is also the legal manner of animal identification in the European Union.

When performed at an early age, ear tagging seems to cause little or no discomfort to lambs. However, using tags improperly or using tags not designed for sheep may cause discomfort, largely due to excess weight of tags for other animals.

Castration is performed on ram lambs not intended for breeding, though some shepherds choose to avoid the procedure for ethical, economic or practical reasons. Ram lambs that will either be slaughtered or separated from ewes before sexual maturity are not usually castrated. Docking, which is a shortening—not a complete removal—of sheep's tails is practiced for health reasons. The tail is removed just below the lamb's caudal tail flaps.

Though docking is often considered cruel and unnatural by animal rights activists, it is considered by sheep producers large and small alike to be a critical step in maintaining the health of sheep. Long, wooly tails make shearing more difficult, interfere with mating, and make sheep extremely susceptible to parasites, especially those that cause flystrike. In Chuck Wooster's *Living with Sheep*, the author anecdotally relates his shearer's response when told of his opposition to docking: "There's nothing natural about a sheep walking around with a dozen pounds of wool on it, and nothing natural about a sheep with a wooly tail.

Natural's got nothing to do with it. If lambs are seen walking around with tails covered by maggots and flies, cut the tails off. Both castrating and docking can be performed with several different instruments. An elastrator places a tight band of rubber around an area, causing it to atrophy and fall off in a number of weeks. This process is bloodless and does not seem to cause extended suffering to lambs, who tend to ignore it after several hours. In addition to the elastrator, a Burdizzo, emasculator, heated chisel or knife are sometimes used. After one to three days in the lambing jugs, ewes and lambs are usually sufficiently stabilized to allow reintroduction to the rest of the flock.

Health

Sheep may fall victim to chemical, pathogenic and physical means of sickness and injury. As a prey species, a sheep's system is designed to hide the obvious signs of illness as much as possible, in order to prevent being targeted by predators. However, there are some signs of ill health that can be ascertained without any special testing. Sick sheep may be unwilling to eat, vocalize excessively, and be generally listless. Throughout history, much of the money and labour of sheep husbandry has gone in to dealing with sheep ailments in order to avoid the heavy losses sustained from them.

Shepherds in history often created remedies through experimentation on the farm. In some countries, sheep do not have the economic impact to necessitate often expensive clinical studies designed to approve drugs specifically for usage with sheep. In such instance, many shepherds resort to extra–label usage of drugs approved for other animals.

In the 20th and 21st centuries, a minority of sheep owners have turned to alternative treatments such as homeopathy, herbalism and even traditional Chinese medicine to treat sheep veterinary problems. Despite some favourable anecdotal evidence from sheep producers, the effectiveness of alternative veterinary medicine has been met with skepticism in scientific journals. The need for traditional anti–parasite drugs and antibiotics is widespread, and is a primary impediment to certified organic farming with sheep.

Many breeders take a variety of preventative measures to ward off problems before they arrive. The first is to ensure that all sheep purchased for the initial flock and replacement animals are healthy to begin with. Many buyers avoid outlets which are known to be clearing houses for animals culled from healthy flocks as either sick or simply inferior. This can also mean maintaining a closed flock, and quarantining new sheep for a month. Two fundamental preventative programmes are maintaining good nutrition and stressing sheep as little as possible.

Handling sheep in loud, erratic ways causes them to emit cortisol, a stress hormone. Elevated amounts of cortisol can lead to a weakened immune system, thus making sheep far more vulnerable to disease. Signs of stress in sheep include: excessive panting, teeth grinding, restless movement, wool eating, and wood chewing. Preventing the presence of harmful chemical agents is also an important part of a sheep owner's work. Common culprits of poisoning include pesticide sprays, inorganic fertilizer, motor oil, as well as radiator coolant (the ethylene glycol antifreeze in this is sweet-tasting).

A common form of preventative medication for sheep are vaccinations and treatments for parasites. Both external and internal parasites are the most prevalent malady in sheep, and impede the productivity of flocks even if they are not fatal. Various worms comprise most of the internal parasites, which are ingested during grazing, incubate within the sheep, and are expelled through the digestive system (beginning the cycle again).

Oral parasite medicines known as drenches are given to a flock to treat worms, sometimes after a count of eggs in the sheep's feces has been taken to assess infestation levels. Afterwards, sheep may be moved to a new pasture to prevent ingesting the same parasites. External sheep parasites include: lice, sheep keds, nose bots, sheep itch mite, and maggots. Keds are blood-sucking parasites that can cause general malnutrition and decreased productivity, but are not fatal. Maggots are those of the bot fly and the blowfly.

Fly maggots cause the extremely destructive condition of flystrike. Flies lay their eggs in wounds or wet, manure-soiled wool, and when the maggots hatch they burrow in to a sheep's living flesh, eventually resulting in death if unchecked. In addition to other treatments, crutching (shearing wool from a sheep's rump) is a common preventative method. Nose bots are flies that inhabit a sheep's sinuses, causing breathing difficulties and discomfort. Common signs are a discharge from the nasal passage, sneezing, and frantic movement such as head shaking. External parasites may be controlled through the use of backliners, sprays or immersive treatments (sheep dips). A wide array of diseases caused by bacteria affect sheep, but a few are especially prevalent and some may even be transmittable to humans. Diseases of the hoof, such as foot rot and foot scald may occur, and are treated with footbaths and other remedies. These painful conditions cause lameness and retard a sheep's ability to feed. Ovine Johne's Disease is a wasting disease that affects young sheep. Blue tongue disease is an insect-borne illness causing fever and inflammation of the mucous membranes.

Soremouth (also known as scabby mouth, contagious ecthyma or orf) is a skin disease leaving lesions that can be transmitted to persons handling infected flocks. More seriously, the organisms that can cause spontaneous enzootic abortion in sheep are easily transmitted to pregnant women. Also of concern are scrapie and foot and mouth disease, as both can decimate entire flocks. The latter poses a significant risk to humans. During the 2001 outbreak of foot and mouth disease, hundreds of sheep in the U.K. were culled, and some rare British breeds were at risk for extinction from the pandemic.

Predation

Other than parasites and disease, predation is a threat to sheep health and thereby the profitability of sheep raising. Sheep have very little ability to defend themselves, even when compared with other prey species kept as livestock. Even if sheep are not directly bitten or survive an attack, they may die from panic or from injuries sustained. However, the impact of predation varies dramatically with region.

In Africa, Australia, the Americas, and parts of Europe and Asia predators can be a serious problem. In contrast, some nations are virtually devoid of sheep predators. Many islands that are known for extensive sheep husbandry are suitable largely because of their predator-free status. Worldwide, canids—including the domestic dog—are responsible for the majority of sheep deaths.

224,200 sheep were killed by predators in 2004, comprising approximately 37 per cent of all ovine deaths for that year. The sheep lost in that year represented a sum total of 18.3 million dollars for sheep producers. Coyotes were responsible for 60.5 per cent of all deaths, with the next largest being domestic dogs at 13.3 per cent. Other North American predators of sheep included cougars (5.7 per cent), bobcats (4.9 per cent), eagles (2.8 per cent), bears (3.8 per cent), and foxes (1.9 per cent). Wolves, ravens, vultures, and other animals together made up the remaining 7.1 per cent of deaths.

As all NASS statistics on sheep only take into account sheep after docking, the American Sheep Industry Association estimates that an additional 50-60,000 lambs were killed (before docking) that were not a part of the count. The number of sheep lost to predators may also be higher when considering that reports are generally only made when there is a reasonable expectation that a producer will be financially reimbursed for the loss.

The only widespread potential predators of sheep are cougars and jaguars, both of which are known to prey on livestock regularly. South American canids such as the Maned wolf and foxes of the genus *Pseudalopex* are also blamed for sheep deaths, but no evidence for a statistically significant amount of predation by these species has ever been presented. Though large, the South African sheep industry is significantly hindered by the innumerable predators present in the country. Other African nations that rely on sheep face a similar problem.

The main Australian predator of sheep is the dingo, which is a large-enough danger to sheep to precipitate the construction of the world's largest fence: the Dingo Fence. In contrast, New Zealand has no large carnivores whatsoever. The sole animal known to attack sheep in New Zealand is the rare, unusual kea parrot endemic to the country's South Island. The U.K. and Ireland once both had wolves and bears, but today only the Red fox and birds of prey remain a tangible threat to sheep in the British Isles.

Sheep producers have used a wide variety of measures to try and combat predation throughout history. Pre-modern shepherds had only the most basic of tools: their own presence and livestock guardian dogs. Whereas sheepdogs herd sheep, guardian dogs are trained to integrate in to flocks and protect them from predators. The ability of these dogs to do so is a transference of the canine pack social structure on to a flock. Following their invention, the focus in dealing with predators shifted to the nearly exclusive use of guns, traps, and poisons to kill predators both defensively and preemptively.

The population of predator species plummeted worldwide, pushing some to extinction or significantly reducing their original ranges. With the appearance of the environmental and conservation movements, and subsequent state, provincial, national and international legislation, simply exterminating predator species failed to be a viable option for protecting flocks.

While killing predators caught directly in the act of attacking sheep may be legal, hunting predators is usually not. Poisons, such as compound 1080 and sodium cyanide, that were previously either placed in bait or in special sheep collars are now banned or restricted in most countries.The 1970s saw an ensuing resurgence in the use of livestock guardian dogs and the development of new methods of predator control, many of them non–lethal. Donkeys and llamas have been used since the 1980's in sheep operations, using the same basic principle as livestock guardian dogs.

Donkeys and llamas—which have a natural dislike of all canines—need no special training to deter predators. However, intact males may kill ewes by attempting to breed them, and must be kept without others of their kind in order to bond with the sheep. Dogs, even those from specialized breeds, need some training to be effective and can be used in concert with other dogs. Dogs are the only guardian animal known to be effective with bears and cougars; donkeys and llamas are usually ineffective as they are themselves vulnerable to predation by bears and cougars.

However, dogs have been killed by wolves and may even attract wolf packs. Whatever species is used for guarding, individual animals may be temperamentally ill–suited to working with sheep. In addition to animal guardians, contemporary sheep operations may use non–lethal predator deterrents such as motion–activated lights and noisy alarms. While these devices have been shown to be successful, predators can become habituated to them.

Sheep were among the first animals to be domesticated by mankind, with sources providing a domestication date between nine and eleven thousand years ago in Mesopotamia. The species has several characteristics—such as a relative lack of aggression, a manageable size, early sexual maturity, a social nature, and high reproduction rates—that made it particularly amenable to taming.

Today, *Ovis aries* is an entirely domesticated animal that is largely dependent on man for its health and survival. Small feral populations of sheep exist, but exclusively in areas that are devoid of predators (usually islands). No feral sheep population has ever reached the scale of feral horses, goats, pigs, or dogs.

Determining the exact genetic relation of domestic sheep to its wild ancestors is a complex problem, and no particular lineage has received complete acceptance in the scientific community. The most common theory currently supported by DNA analysis indicates that *Ovis aries* is jointly descended from both the European (*O. musimon*) and Asiatic (*O. orientalis*) species of mouflon.

It has also been proposed that the European mouflon is an ancient breed of domestic sheep turned feral rather than an ancestor, the lack of a fossil record for the species may support this hypothesis. The urial (*O. vignei*) was once often thought to have been a forebear of domestic sheep; they occasionally interbreed with mouflon in the Iranian part of their range.

However, both the urial, argali, and snow sheep possess a different number of chromosomes than other Ovis species, making any direct influence highly implausible. Contemporary evaluations of sheep DNA show no evidence of urial ancestry. DNA analysis comparing European and Asian breeds of sheep shows a significant percentage of genetic variance between the two. Two explanations for this phenomenon have been posited.

The first is that there is a currently unknown species or subspecies of wild sheep that contributed to the formation of domestic sheep. A second theory suggests that this variation is the result of multiple waves of capture from wild mouflon, similar to the known development of other livestock.

Initially, sheep were kept solely for meat, milk and skins. Archaeological evidence from statuary found at sites in Iran suggests that selection for wooly sheep may have began circa 6000 BC, but the earliest woven wool garments have only been dated to two to three thousand years later. By that span of the Bronze Age, sheep with all the major features of modern breeds were widespread throughout Western Asia. However, one chief difference between ancient sheep and most modern breeds is the technique by which wool could be collected.

Primitive sheep cannot be shorn, and must have their wool plucked out by hand in a process called "rooing".

This is due to the fact that their kemps are still longer than the soft fleece. The fleece may also be collected from the field after it falls out. This trait survives today in unrefined breeds such as the Soay. The Soay, along with other Northern European breeds with short tails, unshearable fleece, diminutive size, and horns in both sexes, are more closely related to ancient sheep than most breeds found today. Originally, weaving and spinning wool was a handicraft practiced at home, rather than an industry.

Egyptians, Babylonians, Sumerians, and Persians all depended on sheep; and though linen was the first fabric to be fashioned in to clothing, wool was a prized product. The raising of flocks for their fleece was one of the earliest industries, and flocks were a medium of exchange in barter economies.

From Southwest Asia, sheep husbandry spread quickly in to Europe. Practically from its inception, ancient Greek civilization relied on sheep as primary livestock, and were even said to name individual animals. Scandanavian sheep of a type seen today—with short tails and multi-coloured fleece—were also present early on. Later, the Roman Empire kept sheep on a wide scale, and the Romans were an important agent in the spread of sheep raising throughout the continent.

Pliny the Elder, in his Natural History (*Naturalis Historia*), speaks at length about sheep and wool. Declaring "Many thanks, too, do we owe to the sheep, both for appeasing the gods, and for giving us the use of its fleece.", he goes on to detail the breeds of ancient sheep and the many colours, lengths and qualities of wool. Romans also pioneered the practice of blanketing sheep, in which a fitted coat (today usually of nylon) is placed over the sheep to improve the cleanliness and luster of its wool.

During the Roman occupation of the British Isles, a large wool processing factory was established in Winchester, England circa 50 AD. By 1000 AD, England and Spain were recognized as the epicenters of sheep production in the

Western world. As the original breeders of the fine-wooled merino sheep that have historically dominated the wool trade, the Spanish gained great wealth. Wool money largely financed Spanish rulers and thus the voyages to the New World by conquistadors.

The powerful *Mesta* (its full title was *Honrado Concejo de la Mesta,* the Honourable Council of the Mesta) was a corporation of sheep owners mostly drawn from Spain's wealthy merchants, Catholic clergy and nobility that controlled the merino flocks. By the Seventeenth century, the *Mesta* held in upwards of two million head of merino sheep.

These flocks followed a seasonal pattern of transhumance across Spain. In the spring, they left the winter pastures (*invernaderos*) in Extremadura and Andalusia to graze on their summer pastures (*agostaderos*) in Castile, returning back again in the autumn. Spanish rulers eager to increase wool profits gave extensive legal rights to the *Mesta,* often to the detriment of local peasantry. The huge merino flocks had a lawful right of way for their migratory routes (*cañadas*). Towns and villages were obliged by law to let the flocks graze on their common land, and the Mesta had its own sheriffs which could summon offending individuals to its own tribunals.

Exportation of merinos was also a punishable offense that required royal permission, thus ensuring a near-absolute monopoly on the breed until Napoleon's invasion of that country in the mid-18th century. After the breaking of the export ban, fine wool sheep began to be distributed worldwide. The export to Rambouillet by Louis XVI in 1786 formed the basis for the modern Rambouillet breed. After the Napoleonic Wars and the global distribution of the once-exclusive Spanish stocks of Merinos, sheep raising in Spain reverted to hardy coarse-wooled breeds such as the Churra, and was no longer of international economic significance.

The sheep industry in Spain was an instance of migratory flock management, with large homogenous flocks ranging over the entire nation. Comparatively, the ovine model used in England was quite different but had a similar importance to economy of the British Empire. Up until the early 20th century, owling (the smuggling of sheep or wool out of the country) was a punishable offense, and to this day the Lord Speaker of the House of Lords sits on a bench known as the Woolsack.

The high concentration and more sedentary nature of shepherding in the U.K. allowed sheep especially adapted to their particular purpose and region to be raised, thereby giving rise to an exceptional variety of breeds in relation to the land mass of the country. This greater variety of breeds also produced a valuable variety of products to compete with the superfine wool of Spanish sheep.

The growth of the sheep industry in Britain quickened in the 15th and 16th centuries due to booming wool prices and the greater pasture available due to a diminished population (the result of the Black Death). More landholders were willing and able to turn their lands over to pasture for sheep, and an influx of Flemish immigrants skilled in cloth making and dyeing during the reign of Edward III helped to cement the wool trade.

By this time, Britain began moving from an open field system to one of enclosure. The unilateral closing of commons by landed gentry had enormously detrimental effects on local communities—entire villages were sometimes depopulated to make way for pasture—and was widely protested. By the time of Elizabeth I's rule, sheep and wool trade was the primary source of tax revenue to the Crown of England.

An important event not only in the history of domestic sheep, but of all livestock, was the work of Robert Bakewell in the 1700s. Before his time, breeding for desirable traits was often based on chance, with no scientific process for selection of breeding stock. Bakewell established the principles of selective breeding—especially line breeding—in his work with sheep, horses and cattle, and his theories were an influence on the subsequent work of Gregor Mendel and Charles Darwin. His most important contribution to sheep was the development of the Leicester Longwool, a quick-maturing breed of blocky conformation that formed the basis for many vital modern breeds.

Today, the sheep industry in the U.K. has diminished

significantly. Even the British taste for mutton (lamb is still popular) has declined, which prompted the creation of the Mutton Renaissance Campaign by the Prince of Wales.

No ovine species native to the Americas has ever been domesticated, despite being closer genetically to domestic sheep than many Asian and European species, having the same number of chromosomes. The first domestic sheep—most likely of the Churra breed—arrived with Christopher Columbus' second voyage in 1493. The next Transatlantic shipment to arrive was with Hernán Cortés in 1519, landing in Mexico. No export of wool or animals is known to have occurred from these populations.

However, Churras were introduced to the Navajo tribe of Native Americans, and became a key part of their livelihood and culture. The modern presence of the Navajo-Churro breed is a result of this heritage. The next transport of sheep to North America was not until 1607 with the voyage of the *HMS Susan Conant* to Virginia. However, the sheep that arrived in that year were all slaughtered because of a famine, and a permanent flock was not to reach the colony until two years later in 1609. Two decades later, the colonists had grown their flock to a total of 400. Sheep were also eventually purchased from the Dutch colonizers of Manhattan.

In 1662, a woolen mill was built in Watertown, Massachusetts, and by the 1640s there were approximately 100,000 head of sheep in the 13 colonies. Early on, the British government banned further export of sheep to the Americas, or wool from it, in an attempt to stifle any threat to the wool trade in the British Isles. One of many restrictive trade measures that precipitated the American Revolution, the sheep industry in the Northeast grew despite the bans.

Gradually throughout the 1900s, sheep production moved westward, and today the vast majority of flocks reside on Western range lands. During this westward migration of the industry, competition between sheep and cattle operations grew more heated, eventually erupting in to range wars. Other than simple competition for grazing and water rights, cattlemen believed that the secretions of the foot glands of sheep made cattle unwilling to graze on places where sheep had stepped.

Another effect of the westward movement of sheep flocks in North America was the decline of wild species such as Bighorn sheep. Most diseases of domestic sheep are transmittable to wild ovines, and such diseases, along with overgrazing and habitat loss, are named as primary factors in the plummeting numbers of wild sheep. Sheep production peaked in the United States during 1940s and 50s at more than 55 million head. Henceforth and continuing today, the number of sheep in North America has steadily declined with wool prices and the lessening American demand for sheep meat.

In South America, especially in Argentina, Chile, Brazil, Uruguay, and Peru, there is an active modern sheep industry. Sheep keeping was largely introduced through immigration to the continent by Spanish and British peoples, for whom sheep were a major industry during the period. South America today has a large number of sheep, but the highest-producing nation kept only just over 15 million head in 2004, far less than most centers of sheep husbandry.

Brazil is, however, not an export nation of any consequence in the sheep industry and sheep operations often find themselves in stiff competition from the immense cattle industry in the country. The most influential region internationally is that of Patagonia, and Patagonian shepherds are often employed by U.S. sheep producers. With few predators and almost no grazing competition, the region is prime land for sheep raising. The most exceptional area of production is surrounding the La Plata river in the Pampas region.

Sheep production in Patagonia peaked in 1952 at more than 21 million head, but has steadily fallen to less then ten today. Most operations focus on wool production for export from Merino and Corriedale sheep; the economic sustainability of wool flocks has fallen with the drop in prices, while the cattle industry continues to grow.

Australia and New Zealand are crucial players in the contemporary sheep industry, and sheep are an iconic part of both countries' culture and economy. New Zealand has the highest density of sheep per capita (sheep outnumber the human population 12–1), and Australia is the world's indisputably largest exporter of sheep and cattle. In 2007, New Zealand even declared February 15 their National Lamb Day, an official holiday celebrating the country's history of sheep production. The First Fleet brought the initial population of 70 sheep from the Cape of Good Hope to Australia in 1788.

The next shipment was of 30 sheep from Calcutta and Ireland in 1793. All of the early sheep brought to Australia were exclusively used for the dietary needs of the penal colonies. The beginnings of the Australian wool industry were due to the vision and efforts of Captain John Macarthur. At Macarthur's urging 16 Spanish merinos were imported in 1797, effectively beginning the Australian sheep industry. By 1801 Macarthur had 1,000 head of sheep, and in 1803 he exported 245 lbs (111 kg) of wool to England. Today, Macarthur is generally thought of as the father of the Australian sheep industry.

The growth of the sheep industry in Australia was explosive. In 1820, the continent held 100,000 sheep, a decade later it had one million. By 1840, New South Wales alone kept 4 million sheep; flock numbers grew to 13 million in a decade. While much of the growth in both nations was due to the active support of Britain in its desire for wool, both worked independently to develop many new high-production breeds: the Corriedale, Coolalee, Coopworth, Perendale, Polwarth, Booroola Merino, Peppin Merino, and Poll Merino were all created in New Zealand or Australia.

Wool production was a fitting industry for colonies far from their home nations. Before the advent of fast air and maritime shipping, wool was one of the few viable products that was not subject to spoiling on the long passage back to British ports. The abundant new land and milder winter weather of the region also aided the growth of the Australian and New Zealand sheep industries.

Flocks in Australia have always been largely range bands on fenced land, and are aimed at production of superfine wool for clothing and other products as well as meat. New Zealand flocks are kept in a fashion similar to English ones, in fenced holdings without herders. Though wool was once the primary income source for New Zealand sheep owners, today it has shifted to meat production.

The Australian sheep industry is the only sector of the industry to receive strident international criticism for its practices. The practice of mulesing, in which skin is cut away from an animal's perineal area without anesthesia to prevent cases of flystrike, has been condemned widely as painful and unnecessary. In response, a programme of phasing out mulesing is currently being implemented.

Most of the sheep meat exported from Australia are either frozen carcasses to the U.K. or live animals to the Middle East. Shipped on converted oil tankers in what has been called crowded, unsafe conditions by critics, live sheep are desired by Middle Eastern nations to meet the requirements ritual halal slaughter. Opponents of the export—such as PETA—say that sheep exported to countries outside the jurisdiction of Australia's animal cruelty laws are treated with horrendous brutality and that halal facilities exist within Australia to make export of live animals redundant. A few celebrities and companies have pledged to boycott all Australian sheep products in protest.

Economic Importance

Domestic sheep have been important to many economies, given that sheep provide a wide array of raw materials. Wool continues to be a vital textile, although in the late 20th century wool prices began to fall dramatically as the result of the popularity and cheap prices for synthetic fabrics. For many shepherds, the cost of shearing is greater than the possible profit from the fleece, making subsisting on wool production alone practically impossible without farm subsidies. Fleeces are used as material in making alternative products such as Wool insulation. In the 21st century, the sale of meat is the most profitable enterprise in the sheep industry.

Sheepskin is likewise used for making clothes, footwear,

rugs, and other products. Byproducts from the slaughter of sheep are also of value: sheep tallow was once used in candlemaking, sheep bone and cartilage has been used to furnish carved items such as dice and buttons as well as rendered glue and gelatin.

Sheep intestine can be formed into sausage casings, and lamb intestine has especially been formed into surgical sutures, as well as strings for musical instruments and tennis rackets. Sheep droppings have even been sterilized and mixed with traditional pulp materials to make paper. Of all sheep byproducts, perhaps the most valuable is lanolin: the waterproof, fatty substance found naturally in sheep's wool and used as a base for innumerable cosmetics and other products.

In the modern era, sheep retain considerable importance in the economies of several countries. Countries such as China, India, Iran and Sudan have extremely large flocks that are generally of national and regional importance. Australia, New Zealand and other countries focus on global exports. Sheep play a major role in the economies of several smaller countries, where the number of sheep may not be great and impact on the global economy is negligible, but is still important locally. Such flocks may be a part of subsistence agriculture rather than a system of trade.

As Food

Sheep meat and milk were one of the earliest staple proteins consumed by human civilization after the transition from hunting and gathering to agriculture. Sheep meat prepared for food is known as either mutton or lamb. "Mutton" is derived from the Old French "*moton*", which was the word for sheep used by the Anglo-Norman rulers of much of the British Isles in the Middle Ages.

This became the name for sheep meat in English, while the Old English word *sceap* was kept for the live animal (eventually forming the word English speakers use today). More recently, "mutton" has been limited to the meat of older sheep; "lamb" is used for that of younger ones, usually those under a year old.

In the 21st century, the nations with the highest consumption of sheep meat are the Persian Gulf states, New Zealand, Australia, Greece, Uruguay, the United Kingdom and Ireland. These countries eat between 14 and 39 lbs. (approximately 3 to 18 kg) of sheep meat per capita, per annum. By comparison, countries such as the U.S. consume only a pound or less (under 0.5 kg). In addition, such countries rarely eat mutton, and may even restrict their habits to the more expensive cuts of lamb: mostly the chop and the leg.

In those that do favour sheep meat, it is often the product of a past history of sheep production, even if they produce little or no sheep today. In such countries in particular, dishes comprising alternative cuts and offal may be popular or traditional. Sheep testicles—called animelles or lamb fries in culinary terminology—are considered a delicacy in many parts of the world. Perhaps the most infamous dish of sheep meat is the Scottish haggis, composed of a sheep's heart, liver and lungs cooked within its stomach.

Though it may have been in antiquity, sheep's milk is no longer drunk directly on any appreciable level. Sheep's milk is, however, valuable in the creation of some popular varieties of cheese and yogurts. Containing 6 per cent fat and double the solids of cow's milk, it can be crafted in to such dairy products with relative ease. Well-known sheep milk cheeses include the Roquefort of France, the Brocciu of Corsica, Manchego from Spain, the Pecorino Romano of Italy and Feta of Greece. Sheep milk does contain 4.8 per cent lactose, which may affect those who are intolerant.

Though not common model organisms, sheep have had played a small, yet influential role in scientific experimentation. Sheep are generally too large and dissimilar to humans to make ideal research subjects, but the few contemporary instances of sheep experimentation has caused a significant impact on science and culture at large. In particular, the Roslin Institute of Edinburgh, Scotland used sheep for genetics research that produced groundbreaking results. In 1995, two ewes named Megan and Morag were the first mammals cloned from differentiated cells.

A year later, a Finnish Dorset sheep named Dolly was the first mammal ever to be cloned from an adult somatic cell. Following this, Polly and Molly were the first mammals to be simultaneously cloned and transgenic.

In the 21st century, controversy raged over a scientific study at the Oregon Health and Science University, which investigated the biological mechanisms producing homosexuality in rams. Organizations such as PETA actively campaigned against the study, accusing scientists of trying to cure homosexuality in the sheep. OHSU and the involved scientists vehemently denied such accusations.

Sheep have had a strong presence within many cultures, especially in areas where they form the most common type of livestock. A wide symbology relates to sheep in art, religion and language. The raising of sheep for wool and meat became a major industry in the U.K. Australia and New Zealand and remains significant. As a result, sheep and sheep shearing have become an important part of the cultural traditions of these countries in particular.

Sheep have become an integral part of many linguistic traditions. In the English language, to call someone a sheep or ovine may allude that they are timid and easily led, if not outright stupid. Male sheep are often used as symbols of virility and power, such as for the St. Louis Rams and the Dodge Ram.

Sheep are key symbols in fables and nursery rhymes like The Wolf in Sheep's Clothing, Little Bo Peep, Baa Baa Black Sheep, and Mary Had a Little Lamb. Novels such as George Orwell's Animal Farm, Philip K. Dick's Do Androids Dream of Electric Sheep? and Thomas Hardy's Far From the Madding Crowd utilize sheep, as either characters or symbols.

The light-hearted detective novel *Three Bags Full* focuses on a flock of anthropomorphic sheep out to solve the murder of their shepherd. Poems like William Blake's "The Lamb", and songs such as Pink Floyd's "Sheep" use sheep for metaphorical purposes. In more modern popular culture, Exploding sheep are a video gaming phenomenon.

The 2007 film *Black Sheep* exploits sheep for horror and

comedic effect, ironically turning sheep into blood-thirsty killers. The Academy Award-winning film *Babe,* adapted from Dick King-Smith's *The Sheep Pig,* revolves around sheep husbandry and utilizes sheep as central characters.

Counting sheep is popularly said to be an aid to sleep, and some ancient systems of counting sheep persist today. Sheep also enter in colloquial sayings and idiom frequently with such phrases as "black sheep".

To call an individual a black sheep implies that they are an odd or disreputable member of a group. This usage derives from the recessive trait which causes an occasional black lamb to be born in to an entirely white flock.

These black sheep were considered undesirable by shepherds, as black wool is not as commercially viable as white wool. Stereotypically, sheep are proverbial for their willingness to follow others of their kind. Citizens who accept overbearing governments have been referred to by the portmanteau neologism of sheeple. Somewhat differently, the adjective "sheepish" is also used to describe embarrassment.

BUFFALOW FARMING

The world's buffaloes are classified into two groups – the Asian and the African. The Asian buffalo is called Bubalus and consists of three species – the anoa of Celebes, the tamaro of Mindori and the arni or Indian wild buffalo. Bubalus bubalis is the name of the domesticated wild Indian buffalo, previously called B. arnee.

There are two general types of the domesticated buffalo, B. bubalis, - the river buffalo and the swamp buffalo. The river buffalo has 50 chromosomes and the swamp type has 48, the amount of genetic material is the same in both. They interbreed and produce fertile progeny with 49 chromosomes. The African buffalo is named Syncerus with a single species S. caffer, with a small number of sub-species. The African buffalo has not been domesticated and will not be discussed further.

The B. Bubalis is widely distributed in Asia, but it has also been introduced to Europe, Near East, China, South America, the former Soviet Union and the Caribbean. The world population of buffaloes is 149 million, of these, 144 million live in Asia. Over half the worlds buffalo population is in India – more than 75 million animals in northern India and Pakistan, buffaloes for milk production have been selected to a large extent.

Swamp Buffaloes

The swamp type is most common in Southeast Asia where it is mostly employed as a draught animal. It has derived its name from the natural habitat which is swamp or marshland. Swamp buffaloes resemble the wild arni in morphological characteristics. Recently, its potential as a meat producer has been discovered. Some strains of the swamp type are larger than others, but there are no distinct breeds. Swamp buffaloes have a very low milk yield and are not used as milk producers. However, crossings between river and swamp buffaloes have been attempted in Thailand, Philippines, Vietnam, and China on a large scale. These crossbred buffaloes are powerful work animals, and produce good quality meat and more milk than the indigenous buffaloes.

River Buffaloes

The river buffalo is the most common type in India, Pakistan, Bulgaria, Hungary, Turkey, Italy and Egypt. They are also found in Brazil and Caucasia. The river buffalo prefers to wallow in clean water and rivers, thereby the name. River buffaloes have been selected for milk production to a larger extent and some river breeds. E.g. Murrah, Nili-Ravi and others are solely used for milk production. India, Pakistan, Italy and Egypt have a widespread culture of consuming buffalo milk. These countries are the most prominent in research on buffaloes.

CURRENT PRACTICE SYSTEMS

Buffaloes are managed under very different conditions over the world. These depend both on the geographic situations and for what purpose the buffaloes are used. Any system from multi-purpose animals kept in backyards to high yielding milk producers in advanced farms exists. Ninety-nine percent of the milk producing buffaloes are owned by small to medium land holding farmers and are merely a source of a small extra income.

One or two buffaloes are a fairly common herd size. The buffaloes are managed under a so called backyard system. They are fed crop resides like wheat straw, paddy straw, sovers, etc. This diet is sometimes supplemented with grazing and/or fodder by the cut-and-carry-system and concentrates. The buffaloes are used as multi-purpose animals and under these conditions; they do not yield large quantities of milk.

In Punjab, northern India, the highest milk consumption in India is noted, approximately 800 grams per capita and day. Here, a well developed milk collection system is in operation through dairy cooperatives. The farms of this area are somewhat bigger than the national average, 10 to 15 buffaloes are common in a family farm. Although cows (cross breeds) are more common, almost all farmers keep a few buffaloes for house hold needs. Mixed farms are also common, where milk from both buffaloes and cattle are produced and sold commercially. At these bigger farms, all green fodder is produced at the farm and the buffaloes are fed a fairly balanced ration of green feed, concentrate and straw.

When a new buffalo is required at the farm, it is usually bought from the market. The buffaloes are often bought in their 2nd or 3rd lactation and sold when they dry off, because they are seen as unproductive animals during this time. There is a very limited system of self recruiting. Calves are neglected and often only used to secure milk let down.

Female calves may get more attention but the reality is that male buffalo calves often starve to death. The calf mortality in India and Pakistan is 30-40 per cent. Milking is predominantly done twice a day by hand. Very few buffalo farmers have so far commenced machine milking, although the number is increasing. Larger farms, such as university and governmental farms contribute little to the total milk production of India and Pakistan. However, the yield per buffalo is higher than in other production systems. Some reasons for this are the better care and feed as well as a larger capital to invest in high yielding buffaloes.

In Caucasia, in the countries of Azerbaijan, Georgia and Armenia, buffaloes are used as multi-purpose animals. In the past, the animals were used for draught mostly. With the mechanization of the agriculture, these animals have lost some of their importance. In Italy and Bulgaria, the buffaloes have been selected for milk and meat production and almost exclusively used as such.

The total population of buffaloes in Italy is 161,000, 100,000 of these are breed able females. In Italy, the majority of buffaloes are kept in herds of up to 50 animals. Machine milking was introduced in the 1960's and is widely used. Twice or even three times milking per day is common practice. Tandem or herring bone parlors in various sizes are common.

The Romanian buffalo is considered to be a breed of its own. It is a Mediterranean type and is sometimes crossed with the Murrah breed. The population is 210,000 animals including 97,000 breed able females. The lactation yield is 900 to 1400 kg and the length is 252-285 days. Twice a day hand milking is practiced at private farms while research and industrial farms using machine milking. Bulgarian farms are often run as cooperatives with 250-500 buffaloes in one farm. They are equipped with machine milking and other technology.

The buffalo population of Turkey is 316,000 animals; approximately half of the population consists of milked females. The production is 600-1000 kg of milk per animal and lactation. The animals are mainly kept in herds of 1 to 15 animals at private farms. Hand milking once or twice a day is the common practice. The buffaloes of Egypt are of a relatively small size and kept for dual purpose such as milk and meat. There are nearly 4 million buffaloes in Egypt and over 95 per cent are kept in small holding farms with one to three buffaloes in a herd. The contribution of buffalo milk to the total milk production in Egypt is 65 per cent.

BEHAVIOUR OF BUFFALOES

The natural behaviour of buffaloes has been studied

amongst the feral buffaloes (Swamp type) of the Northern Territory in Australia. By knowing the natural behaviour of buffaloes, much can be gained when it comes to managing and feeding the animal in the commercial system. Different types of group formations can be seen among feral buffaloes. The strongest is that within a clan.

A clan consists of mothers and their calves; it can also consist of generations of buffaloes. In a clan, all buffaloes are well known to each other. A group consists of a number of clans. In a group, depending on the size, buffaloes may not know each other as well as in a clan. A herd consists of several groups. The clan, group and herd only consist of female buffaloes and male calves up to two or three years of age. At this age, the bulls are driven from the clan and from their own groups. These groups are loose and of different size. Single bulls as well as large bull groups can be seen.

A group of buffaloes share a camp, where they spend the nights. Nearby, but never within a camp is a dung heap. This is the area where buffaloes defecate. At the hottest time of day the buffaloes got to wallow. This is either a mud hole with only little water in it or a larger lagoon or river with deep and clean water. The wallow can be shared by a group or even by a herd, depending on the size of the wallow. In the dry season, females and calves are separate from the bulls. The females and calves gather where there is abundance of water, green feed and shade. Bulls gather in the open plains where the feed is dry. In the beginning of the wet season, the bulls and females merge for breeding.

Buffaloes are considered to be docile and friendly animals. Aggressive behaviour seldom occurs. For example, a new group of buffaloes is allowed to enter another groups' wallow or to drink from their water hole. Buffaloes are a bit dull and slow learners. It takes them a long time to get used to new situations and routines. However, they are easily stressed and may become very nervous if confronted with new situations.

Wallowing Behaviour

Wallowing has two purposes; the most obvious is that of

cooling, the other is protection from insects. Wallowing during daytime is done during the hottest hours. Wallowing during nighttime is instead a way for the animal to protect itself from insects. The buffalo has few sweat glands and a dark skin which makes it difficult for them to maintain their body temperature in hot and humid environments. Wallowing is a very important way for the buffaloes to maintain heir body temperature.

When buffaloes enter the water, they defecate and/or urinate. This seems to be a way to mark their wallow. Wallowing behaviour is a learnt behaviour. An animal that has not wallowed from birth with other animals will not do so on its own. Teaching such an animal to wallow is almost impossible for humans. The buffalo has to learn it from other buffaloes, even so, the adult buffalo will be very suspicious and may not wallow by its own choice. If no water or mud hole is available, the buffaloes behave more like cattle. They will seek shade and graze more during the cool hours and less during the hot hours.

The most important way among buffaloes to communicate is by smell. The buffaloes recognize each other by smelling each other. Smell is used when marking a territory. Buffaloes will rub themselves against trees to leave scent and they defecate to mark their territory. Vocal communication is important especially from calves. There are both friendly and hostile vocal communications. Posture is important when deciding rank and dominance order. A threatening animal will lower and shake its head.

BREEDING BEHAVIOUR

Males and females live in separate groups. They will merge in the beginning of the wet season for mating. The bulls can detect females in heat by their scent and find their camp. There is a period of foreplay before the actual mating takes place. This period is 1 to 3 days and allows the animals to get to know each other. The bull will not leave a female in estrus and he will not allow another bull to come near her. Only the most dominant bulls will mate.

There are very strong bonds between the mother and her calf. If the calf is a male, the bond holds for approximately 2 to 3 years. Thereafter the calf is driven from the clan. In the case of a female calf, the bond exists for life. Shortly before parturition the mother moves away to give birth alone. Within 30 minutes after the calf is born all members of the clan has "inspected" the newborn and touched it with their noses. Nearly all members of the group have come from this inspection. This inspection seems to serve as an introduction of the newly born. It also facilitates adoption of the calf if the mother should die. Adoptions always occur among buffalos whereas it is hardly seen in other species.

The calf walks with its mother as soon as it can stand. This behaviour is different from cattle where the cow leaves its calf to go grazing. Nursing of the calves is common among buffaloes. The calves are left with a "care-taking-animal" who is often a female, but seldom a young bull. The other females go away to graze and leave their calves. Should there be a threat to the calves, they will simply call and their mothers will come running to their aid.

REPRODUCTION AND BREEDING

Buffaloes are said to be seasonal breeders. However, this is a simplification of the truth. Buffaloes are polyestral animals and may breed all year round. Both males and females are sensitive to heat stress and to changes in nutrition. These factors contribute to a lesser frequency of breeding and conception rate in the summer time.

The domesticated river buffalo is divided into several breeds. The most important in milk production in India is the Murrah breed. The Murrah originates from the area around Delhi. From that area it has been spread to other parts of India. The breeds Surti and Nili-Ravi are believed to have developed from the Murrah through geographical isolation. The Nili-Ravi buffaloes were two different breeds (Nili and Ravi) but are now considered to be a single breed.

The Kundi breed is also of importance in the milk production. Traditionally the breeds of Europe have been of the local Mediterranean type and the breeds of Caucasia, the Caucasian type. The most important breed of Bulgaria is the Bulgarian Murrah, which is the result of the cross breeding between the local Mediterranean buffaloes and the Indian Murrah followed by upgrading with Indian Murrah. Cross breeding the local buffaloes with high yielding elite buffaloes has not started in several countries.

Bulls reach sexual maturity at 2 to 3 years of age. Semen is produced all year round but it is highly affected by heat stress and low quality feed. The buffalo bull seems to be most fertile in spring when the volume of ejaculate and the sperm concentration is the highest. The vitality of the sperms are also much higher in spring than other times of the year. Corresponding values are lowest in summer time. Heat stress may have a negative effect on libido.

Wild or feral female buffaloes reach sexual maturity at 2 to 3 years of age. Domesticated buffaloes that are cared for and fed properly may reach puberty earlier. Puberty is highly affected by management factors. Size is more important than age and a Murrah heifer should weigh around 325 kg at insemination or mating and 500 kg at her first calving. The estrus cycle varies between 21 and 29 days depending on breed.

The total duration of estrus is usually 24 hours but varies between 12-72 hours. The most reliable sign of estrus is frequent urination. The signs are much less pronounced than in cattle. Many buffaloes show estrus only at night time, and then it is difficult to detect. A lactating animal may have a slight decrease in milk yield when in heat, although it is seldom as pronounced as in cattle. The buffalo may be more restless and be difficult to milk.

Buffaloes, generally, have more difficulty conceiving when using artificial insemination than cattle do. Reports from NDRI, Karnal, India, shows that the conception rate for first insemination is around 40.per cent and the conception rate for third insemination is around 77 per cent. The gestation period for buffaloes averages 308 to 318 days. The age of the heifer at her first calving is usually around 37-40 months (3 to 3.5 years).

The first post partum heat varies greatly with season, breed and individual. It has been reported to appear within less than 60 days in some cases and over 230 in others. Average post partum estrus in the Murrah breed of India has been reported to be 100 days. The first post partum estrus is not always fertile, especially if it comes very near partus.

Breeding

In order to achieve a high lifetime milk production, regularity in conception and a short calving interval are the most important factors. The female must be serviced soon after the calving in order to conceive. Having a breeding bull with the dams all the time enhances the chances of fertile mating. This bull seldom misses a female in heat. However, to be able to calculate the time of calving it is advisable to keep some sort of record of expected heat. The observant farmer will soon learn how his buffaloes behave when in heat and when to expect conception and calving. The females can be teased with a bull twice a day around expected estrus.

A breeding bull can be put into service from 3 years of age. In Italy, it is recommended that a breeding bull on a large farm should be exchanged after a maximum of 5 years. One bull, if managed correctly, can serve 20 to 25 females. In a smaller farm, the bull should be exchanged more often to avoid interbreeding. If the bull shows signs of loss of interest in the females or is otherwise ill, he should be taken out of service immediately. In order to perform best, the bulls must be fed high quality feed and be protected from heat and cold stress in the same ways as the rest of the herd. Bulls should not be used for service more than twice a week.

Calving interval is highly dependable on season of breeding, farm and year and can therefore be shorter in some farms while longer in others. In order to shorten the calving interval the female should be serviced again as soon as possible after calving.

Weaning of calves at birth has shown to decrease the service period compared to unweaned buffaloes. A shorter service period will lead to a shorter calving interval a calving interval of less than 410 days is recommended. Although intensive research is going on at various universities and institutions around the world, breeding programmes for buffaloes are not readily available for the common farmer. In the state of Gujarat in India, the National Dairy Development Board has a breed improvement programme called Dairy Herd Improvement Programme Actions (DIPA).

The genetic gain of the buffaloes are being increased through selection of sires to breed sires and dams to breed sires. A progeny testing programme is being followed producing 100 completed first lactation records of progeny per bull. 20 bulls are put to test every year, 2000 doses of frozen semen from each bull is being distributed to the selected villages and 5000 doses are stored until the test results are available.

By replacing good milking buffaloes with their own daughters instead of purchasing new buffaloes from the market some advantages are gained. Firstly, spreading of diseases is limited compared to selling and purchasing on the market. Secondly, the farmer has full control over his herd. He knows the heritage of each buffalo and can make more accurate decisions concerning the future. He will know whether the buffalo has had any diseases or problems with fertility. The buffaloes will get to know the farmer and are therefore easier to handle, which is most important when it comes to machine milking.

High milk yield, ease to milk, short let down time, high conception rate and temperament are some of the selection criteria which are desirable in a good breeding buffalo. When creating a breeding programme it is important to keep records of the buffaloes.

Heritage, milk yield of mother, peak yield, lactation length, services per conception are parameters that are important to keep track of. When breeding for a higher milk yield it is especially important to register the milk production correctly at regular intervals. The International Committee for Animal Recording (ICAR) has put up some basic rules for milk recording which are similar in all countries:

OVERALL MANAGEMENT OF THE BUFFALO

Buffaloes should be cared for as the valuable live capital they are. By proper management buffalo farming is indeed profitable. By deciding at birth whether a calf should be a milk producer or not, proper care of the calves is easier and less costly. The farmer can then focus on the future milk producers and cull the others. No matter how good the genetic potential, no animal will perform satisfactory if it is not cared for and fed properly.

Bull calves after high yielding dams can be bred at the farm for future breeding of the females. They can be sold to breeding stations for progeny-testing.

HEALTH CONTROL

The buffaloes should be checked daily for injuries and illnesses. Wounds and open sores are a perfect growing place for all kinds of bacteria! It is easy to keep control over milking buffaloes since they are closely studied twice a day. But apart from looking at the udder at milking the farmer or milker should observe the whole animal. Not only milking animals need to be checked on, but also heifers, calves and bulls.

Lameness and large injuries are easier to detect than small scratches. Lameness can be caused by injuries in the hooves and legs as well as back pains. By touching the animal all over the body, the location of the injury can be located.

Large as well as small injuries must be taken care of. Bleeding sores may require veterinary attention although this is quite rare. Wounds shall be carefully cleaned. The best is to use clean water and mild soap. Cleaning should be done with clean hands, cloths and very gently. Chemicals, such as ethanol and iodine might hurt. Never attend to wounds during milking! It is best to take the animal to a sick box or undisturbed area and attend the wounds.

Looking at the feces is an easy way to detect internal defects. This is easy in the milking place when one pale of feces can be related to one buffalo. If the feces looks different than usual, the milker / farmer should be observant.

If the buffalo is not eating properly or otherwise seems

dull and "unfit" it might be a sign of some kind of illness. If an animal has some or all of the above mentioned symptoms. It is advisable to measure the rectal temperature. Normal rectal temperature is 38° to 39°C. If it is above that, the animal may have some sort of infection and a veterinarian should be called.

The quicker a wound or an infection is taken care of, the smaller the risk of more buffaloes becoming ill.

Parasites

In the tropics and subtropics, parasites, ticks and mosquitoes can be a big problem. Internal parasites may cause malfunction of the digestive tract and thereby decrease feed utilization. Ticks and mosquitoes cause discomfort and damage to the skin which in turn can lead to inflammatory processes.

Chemicals and drugs to fight parasites should be used both as a profylax and in case it is needed. A disadvantage with chemicals and drugs is that they often leave traces in the milk. Some may be harmless and undetectable, yet others may influence processing of the milk and/or leave traces dangerous for human consumption.

Chemicals against parasites should be sprayed on the animals. Care must be taken not to spray in the eyes or genital area. In the face and around the genitals, a sponge with the chemical should be used. Dip baths, which are widely used for cattle are most unsuitable for buffaloes. The buffaloes will see the dip baths as wallows and this has at least two disadvantages. 1) They may enjoy wallowing in the dip, thus being difficult to get out. This may cause harm to the skin. 2) Buffaloes natural behaviour is to defecate in their wallow, thus making the dip bath extremely unhygienic.

Vaccination Programmes

There are a number of vaccines available for common diseases. Most vaccination programmes are more efficient if applied to the young calf and thereafter given as a booster with regular intervals. This is further evidence of the advantage of recruiting calves at the farm. Buffaloes are sensitive to the same diseases as cattle. The disease strikes harder on animals in poor condition. In order to protect the animals, they should be properly vaccinated and de-wormed at regular intervals. It is important to include all animals at the farm in a veterinary control programme in order to minimize risks of disease out breaks. In Italy, all controlled animals are checked with six months interval for tuberculosis, brucellosis and leukosis. Infected animals are immediately taken out of producition and culled.

FEEDING

Buffaloes are, like cattle, ruminants. This means that they utilize micro-organisms in the rumen to digest the feed. The feed eaten by ruminants are mainly of vegetable origin. The ruminant is an expert in converting cellulose and other fibrous materials into high quality milk and meat. Their digestive capacity is greater than the non-ruminant. Ruminants "chew the cud" e.g. regurgitate the food to the mouth and chew it several times, thus helping the breakdown.

The feed will enter the rumen compartment when swallowed by the animal. The rumen is an anaerobe environment, e.g. no oxygen is present. The feed is exposed to microbes such as bacteria, protozoa and fungi. These microbes attack the feed particles and by enzymatic action the components are broken down and used for their own metabolism, growth and propagation. The feed is masticated, regurgitated and exposed to microbes in the rumen. Large particles will become smaller and eventually be transported to the reticulum and further on.

How long time a specific feed particle will stay in the rumen depends on size, palatability and fibre content of the feed. The buffalo has slower rumen movement than cattle, which leads to a slower rate of ingesta outflow. The pH of the rumen content is similar to that of cattle, and it is affected in the same manner. Normal pH is between 6 and 7 depending on feed and time of feeding.

The waste end products of the microbial attack are methane and carbon dioxide which are eructated. Volatile fatty acids (VFA) of which acetic, propionic and butyric acids are the predominant ones, are together with ammonia absorbed by the animal through the rumen wall, and transported via the blood to, e.g. the liver and udder where they serve as building material for chemical compounds such as glucose, protein and fat.

Ammonia can be utilised directly by the rumen microbes to synthesize proteins. To be correct, one is actually not feeding the buffalo, but its' microbes. Ruminants are entirely dependent on the function of the rumen microbes. Therefore, it is important to keep the rumen environment healthy. The easiest and best way is to feed a high amount of good quality roughage and a smaller amount of good quality concentrate.

Almost all protein is attacked by the microbes and utilized in their metabolism and incorporated in the microbial mass. Microbial protein is of high quality and is absorbed as amino acids after being digested by gastric enzymes in the abomasum. Ammonia which is absorbed by the rumen wall and transported by the blood to the liver, is converted to urea. In case of protein deficiency, urea can be utilized by the rumen microbes as a non-protein nitrogen source to build protein.

In this way nitrogen is circulated and efficiently used by the animal. Protein can be protected to withstand microbial attack. It is then called "by-pass protein". By-pass protein is only degraded in the abomasum and small intestine where it undergoes enzymatic attack similar to that of mono-gastric animals. By-pass-protein is commercially available in some ready made concentrates and is usually given to high producers.

Carbohydrates are the predominant sources of energy for ruminants. Carbohydrates, or sugars, are the components of starch and fibers. Fibre is a common name for cell-wall components such as cellulose, hemi-cellulose and lignin. Starch can be degraded by animal gastric enzymes, whereas fibers cannot. Ruminants can utilize fibers to a larger extent than mono-gastric animals because of the ruminal microbes. However, lignin (wood-fibre) is not utilized. It is generally believed that buffaloes utilize fibre more efficiently than cattle do. The coefficient of digestion being 5-8 per cent higher in buffaloes than in cattle.

Fat is not as such required in other than very small amounts for the ruminant. However, what ever fat is present in the feed undergoes microbial attack and degradation. Unsaturated fatty acids are hydrolyzed and thus saturated. This is one of the reasons for the milk and body fat of the ruminant to be of equal composition, largely independent of the type of feed given.

If the fat can in some form be protected from ruminal degradation, and instead be utilized in the lower intestinal tract, it may be used as an additional energy source. However, it may then alter the milk fat composition unfavourably. Too much unprotected fat in the diet depresses the ability of the microbes to ferment fibers, thus influencing the energy utilisation negatively.

NUTRIENT REQUIREMENTS

In order to utilize the animal, feed and economical resources as efficiently as possible, one must know the nutrient requirements of the animals. If an animal is wrongly fed this may lead to diseases, loss of production and thereby economical losses.

By knowing what a specific animal needs, proper advice concerning purchase, cultivation and feeding systems can be given. Requirements for buffaloes are more or less the same as for cattle, therefore, nutrient requirement tables for dairy cattle may be used as a guidance, the farmer must observe the animals and change feeding system with the guidance of an extension officer if it seems unsuitable.

Sources of energy are predominantly carbohydrates like fibre and starch and fat to a lesser extent. For buffaloes, fibre in the form of roughage is the most important and cheapest energy source. When calculating feed ratios for buffaloes the term metabolizable energy (ME) is used. This means the amount of energy that can be used by the animal for maintenance, growth, lactation etc. The gross energy (GE) of the feed is the amount present in the feed, when entering the animal, much of the energy is converted into heat which is lost through the thermal regulation. Energy is also lost in the feces and urine as well as in the methane and carbon dioxide gases.

Energy is measured in calories (cal) and joules (J) (1 cal equals 4.18 J). The most common is to use the term Mega calories (Mcal) or Mega joules (MJ) which means a million cal or J. Another measurement is Total Digestible Nutrients (TDN) which is the sum of carbohydrates and fat in the diet. The unit for TDN is kg or gram. The energy ratio in the feed may be increased by adding fat in protected form, thus transferring the digestion from rumen to the intestinal tract. Feeding of protected fat (1 kg safflower oil) has proven to increase nutrient utilization. Feeding of unprotected fat in similar amounts has shown to adversely affect nutrient utilization.

Protein is required for growth, tissue repair and milk production among other things. Good sources of protein are leguminous forage, grain and oil-seed-cakes. The protein requirements are measured in Crude protein (CP) in kg or gram.

Minerals are essential for many body functions. The macro-minerals calcium and phosphorus are especially important in milk production. They are also vital for the skeleton and the function of nerve-impulses. Phosphorus is the mineral included in the body's energy metabolism, ATP. When considering the Ca and P requirements for the animal it is equally important to consider the ratio in which it is given. The Ca:P ration should be 2:1 since there exists and antagonist relationship between the two minerals concerning uptake from the small intestine.

Salt, e.g. sodium and potassium together with chloride are the more important micro-minerals. Minerals are present in various amounts in feed and water. Vitamins are essential for total body function. Most vitamins are synthesized by the animal or it's rumen microbes. Such vitamins, B, C and K (and to some extent D) does not need to be fed.

Vitamin B is synthesized by ruminal microbes, vitamin K by intestinal microbes and vitamin C in the tissues. Vitamin

D is formed when the precursor, found on the skin on animals and on grass, is exposed to UV-rays, in tropical countries deficiency of vitamin D is rare. Vitamins A and E are not synthesized in the animal but must be supplied. Vitamin A is found in silage, fresh grass, dark green leaves, peas and carrots. Cereals are a source of vitamin E.

Mineral and/or vitamin mixture should always be supplied in order to fully meet the requirements. Animals which do not receive a ready made concentrate mixture with mineral and vitamin supplement, must be fed supplement in the form of "lick stones" of which the animals have free access to or as "powder" fed once or twice a day individually. Vitamins may be included in the mineral feed, but vitamins are more sensitive and may be destroyed if kept in sunlight. Care must therefore be taken to store vitamin supplements correctly.

Water

Water is essential for most body functions, such as body temperature control, milk production and maintaining blood plasma volume. Thermal regulation of the animal is the most water consuming process. The animal receives water in three different ways

- Drinking water
- Water in feed
- Metabolic water = water made from feed degradation

Drinking water is the most important water source and should be of good hygienic quality. The water available in feed is highly dependent on the dry matter in feed. Straw, hay and cereals include little water, whereas silage and fresh grass may contain as much as 70 percent.

The water requirements of the buffalo depends on;

- The diet (dry matter)
- The environment (humidity, temperature)
- Physiological function (growth, pregnancy, lactation etc.)

Generally, buffaloes require more water than cattle under the same circumstances and should have access to clean cool water ad libitum. A restricted water intake leads to a decrease in dry matter intake and thus affects milk production and growth negatively. Salinity of water is seldom a problem in dairy buffalo feeding. A salt content of up to 5 g/liter of water can be used for buffaloes. However, temporary diarrhea may be caused by water approaching the higher levels.

The main diet for the buffalo is roughage such as grass, legumes and straw. The roughage can be fed either fresh as pasture or in a cut-and-carry-system, or conserved as hay or silage. The roughage is often complemented with grains, concentrate and agro-industrial by-products such as oil-seed cakes, sugar cane tops etc. The roughage should form the base of the feed ration and contribute to meet (at least) the total maintenance requirements.

Grains and concentrate should be fed only to meet additional requirements such as growth, pregnancy and milk production. Too much non-fibrous feed will alter the rumen environment. In the long run this could lead to serious problems in feed digestion causing loss of appetite, weight loss and a drop in milk yield. This is especially important for animals under stress, such as high growth rate and high milk yield. The roughage should be of good quality, both nutritional and hygienic quality, this cannot be emphasized enough.

Types of Roughage

The most common roughage is grass of a number of species. Lucerne, berseem and clover are herbaceous legumes and have an advantage over grass as they are nitrogen fixing. This means that the plants will (with the help of bacteria) fix air-nitrogen and thus they are less dependent on the nitrogen content of the soil. These plants contain more protein than grass under the same circumstances. Lucerne (or Alfalfa) has several advantages. It contains an elevated amount of calcium, vitamin E and caroteen which are of major importance for milk production.

There are also tree legumes which can be used as high quality feed, e.g. Leucaena leucocephala, Gliricida spp., Sesbania and others. As many of the tree legumes contain anti-nutritional compounds which may depress digestibility as well as decrease feed intake, they should not be fed as the sole source of roughage. A maximum ratio of 50 per cent tree legumes in the total diet can be considered as a safe level. Since buffaloes are strict grazers, the trees should be pruned and the branches or leaves given to the buffaloes.

Pruning with regular interval of 6 to 10 weeks increases re-growth of the leaves. Roughage of lesser quality are straws. Straw from rice, barley, wheat, sorghum etc. are widely used in feeding ruminants. Their protein content is zero and their energy content low because of their largely lignified cell-walls. Rice or paddy straw has a high silica content in the cell walls which makes it difficult to digest.

Harvesting Roughage

In the beginning of the growth season, the protein and sugar (energy) content of the grass is high and the lignin content low. Thus, the grass is of high quality. With maturity the protein and sugar content decreases and the cell walls become lignified. The growth pattern is the same for legumes although it is a little slower. It is therefore important to harvest the roughage in the optimal period and to conserve it for use under dry seasons. Pastures should not be over or under grazed. Over grazing leads to insufficient forage in the later season and the soil will be more vulnerable to erosion and permanent damage. In the case of under grazing, the pasture is not utilized efficiently. The grass will grow quicker than the animals can eat. Thus the nutrient composition will change unfavourably to high lignin and low protein content. In many areas, grass is not harvested even if not grazed and is left as "standing hay". However, the standing hay has a very low nutritive quality, close to that of straw.

Chaffing, grinding and pelleting are ways to improve nutritive quality of straws to some extent by making the nutrients available to the rumen microbes. Chemical treatment with alkali or ammonia are effective ways of improving quality. Ammonia treated, chaffed straw may even substitute green forage for low milk producing buffaloes to some extent.

The term concentrate means that a high amount of nutrients are concentrated in a small amount of dry feed. The most typical concentrates for tropical countries are oilseed cakes of different types. Oilseed cakes are the common name for products that are derived of the oil for human use and the remainder is pressed together to form a cake. The cakes have a relatively high energy content but are mostly used because of their very high protein content.

Other types of feed which can be classified as concentrate are molasses and urea. Urea can be used by the microbes as a source of nitrogen. The use of urea also requires an easily fermented energy source for the micro-organisms e.g. molasses. The micro-organisms must always have a good balance between protein and energy in the rumen to be able to do their qualified job. There are a number of ready made concentrates on the market manufactured by various companies. Care should be taken to ensure that the quality of the concentrate is up to standard.

Barley, wheat, oat, rye, maize and sorghum grains are excellent feed for ruminants, given in balanced amounts. However, since they are used for human consumption their use as animal feed is limited.

Voluntary Intake

The definition of voluntary intake is the amount of feed an animal can eat per day. It is commonly expressed in kg of dry matter or in percent of live weight. After having considered the nutrient requirements of the animal and the feed stuff to be used the proper feeding regime can be calculated. However, one must take into consideration how much the animal can eat.

A high producing lactating cow can eat more than a low producing. Similarly a growing heifer may eat more than a dry cow. As pointed out before, feed intake decreases with high environmental temperature and humidity. Individual feeding usually results in higher feed intake due to less competition for feed and a more relaxed atmosphere.

A rough estimation of voluntary intake for a buffalo heifer

is 2.2 to 2.5 per cent of its' live weight per day, if provided with a small portion of straw, a large portion of green feed and some concentrate. A milk producing buffalo should be able to consume good quality feed up to 3 per cent of its' live weight. A too high ratio of straw in the diet reduces voluntary intake. A protein content of less than 6 per cent also reduces intake of that feed.

Practical Feeding of the Lactating Buffalow

Lactating buffaloes should be given the best feed the farm can offer. Producing milk is one of the most energy demanding biological processes. Weight loss is common in high producing animals during the first month of lactation because they can not consume a sufficient amount of energy. A popular term is that the animals are milking off the fat. It is therefore important that the buffalo is in good health status at partus.

Traditional feeding patterns for buffaloes all over the world is subjected to forages and crop production of the season which affects the level of milk production. Forage is insufficient during the dry season and abundant during the rainy season. Shortages are overcome by conserving forages as hay or silage.

Formulating feed ratios for milk producing buffaloes starts with theoretical calculating of the requirements. As there are no standardized international tables for dairy buffaloes' requirements, the calculations here are based on NCR's tables for dairy cattle. It is important to know the buffaloes live weight, this is most accurately done by weighing the animals three times in a week and calculating the average. However, this requires an animal scale and is further very time consuming.

Weighing the animals once is good as a guidance. The milk yield should be known as well as the fat percentage. Recommendations are at least 3 days of milk recording to calculate the average yield and fat percentage. For simplicity, the yield is then calculated to 4 per cent fat corrected milk. The total requirements is gained by summing requirements for maintenance and for milk production.

If the animal seems to be too fat at the time of weighing,

the maintenance requirements may be reduced by 10 per cent. Similarly, if the animal is too skinny, 10 per cent may be added to the maintenance requirements. The feeding regime of the buffaloes can then be decided. Primarily, crops grown on the farm should be included in the diet.

For the optimal economic feeding regimes the feed should be analyzed at a laboratory for dry matter content, energy and crude protein and for calcium and phosphorus. It is important to note that silage should not form the sole source of roughage because its' high amount of easily fermentable carbohydrates and the physical structure which does not realy stimulate rumen contraction.

As a rule of thumb, the amount of silage in a diet should not exceed 30 per cent of the total dry matter intake if concentrate is also given. If the diet is solely made from roughage the silage ration may be increased to 60 per cent. On the other hand, alfalfa hay contains much too much protein and therefore it is important to give a mixture of silage, hay and perhaps straw.

In this example the maintenace requirements can be met by giving 5 kg wheat straw and 5 kg maize silage on a dry matter basis. Alfalfa hay of 2 kg and 8 kg of wheat straw also gives the requirements, however, it is not likely that the buffalo will eat it, because of its texture. We need to provide another 12.85 Mcal for the milk production. This can be provided by increasing the amount of forage if it is of good quality or it may be provided by concentrate. However, the costs for different fodder's should be taken into account, if the farm can produce sufficient forage of good quality it is probably more wise to increase the amount of home grown forage in the diet than by purchasing expensive concentrate.

Only phosphorus needs to be added. The Ca:P ratio should be approximately 2:1 therefore, 22 g P needs to be provided in this diet. It is also clear that the buffalo should be able to produce milk without any concentrate in this example. The total amount of dry matter comes to 14 kg in this example and we had calculated with 16.5 kg. Because of the relatively rough texture of this diet 14 kg DM is probably as much as the buffalo can eat. Including urea in the diet may be a cheap and good way to "help up" a low protein diet. One must remember, however, that a source of highly soluble carbohydrates such as molasses must be included in a urea diet. The maximum level of urea is 25 per cent in the total diet. An alternative is to feed ready made urea-molasses blocks.

Controlling the animals' intake of feed is a good practice. Low yielders tend to eat more than they require and at the same time it is difficult for the high yielders to eat enough. It is therefore vital that the feed is analyzed and the milk yield known, to provide the requirement of each animal.

Feeding of the Calf

Calf mortality is very high, in India it is often 30-40 per cent before 3 months of age, and in Italy the figures may be higher. This is caused by malpractice such as negligence, limited milk feeding, injuries and diseases. By increasing the amount of feed to the calf's requirements and by practicing the following instructions the mortality can be decreased.

Colostrum is the most important and most suitable feed for the newborn calf. It contains all the nutrients needed along with the vital antibodies. It is crucial for the survival of the calf that it receives colostrum during the first 12 hours of its life, the earlier the better. The calves should be given colostrum as long as the mother provides it e.g. 3 to 4 days. Any surplus colostrum can be frozen and then thawed and carefully heated to 39?C. If no freezing facilities are available colostrum can stay fresh for a couple of days if it is cooled in a hygienic container. Colostrum can be fermented with living lactic acid culture. Fermented colostrum can be kept for at least a week and up to two weeks if cooling facilities are available.

If the calf is not allowed to suckle its mother it should be provided with colostrum as soon as possible after birth. If it is not possible to feed the calf directly after milking the buffalo, colostrum should be cooled in order to maintain hygienic quality. Colostrum must never be boiled. By boiling the milk the antibodies are destroyed and hence, cannot be utilized as such by the calf.

The natural eating behaviour of the calf is to suckle its mother often and to consume a small amount of milk at each suckling period. It is best for the calves reared under artificial conditions if their eating behaviour is as "natural" as possible. Colostrum should be fed to the calf at least twice daily with equal intervals.

The calf should be trained to drink from a bucket. The easiest way to do this is to dip clean fingers into the milk and then allow the calf to lick and suck the fingers. The hand is then gradually drawn into the milk in the bucket while the calf is still suckling. Once the calf has learnt to drink it is easy to feed. The calf may need assistance for 5 days.

There are special nipples which can be put in the bucket. The calf will suckle these, hence it will need less assistance from the After the colostrum period, whole milk should be provided to the calf until 15 days of age @ a level of 1/8th to 1/10th of the calf's body weight. Milk replacer can be fed along with the whole milk provided that it has a certain composition of nutrients. It is not advisable to completely substitute whole milk with milk replacer.

Milk and/or replacer should be offered to the calf on at least two occasions per day. The milk and/or replacer should be served at body temperature. At two weeks of age, the calf should be introduced to good quality green feed and concentrates, as a calf starter. This stimulates the rumen to grow and function properly.

An alternative method is to rear calves with foster mothers. In Italy, 40 per cent of the buffalo calves are reared by suckling an old and less productive buffalo or even a cow. This has several advantages, e.g. little labour is required concerning feeding of the calf and the calf will secure it's nutrient intake itself.

Buffalo calves fed with stovers of maize, bajra and oat cannot meet their nutrient requirements and are often in negative energy and protein balance. However, feeding the calves with treated stovers with a urea-molasses-salt complex both enhances the palatability of the stovers as well as the digestibility and nutrient value. Buffalo male calves weighing

150-200 kg has proven to increase the intake of treated stovers verses untreated ones and thereby increasing weight gain, nitrogen balance and health.

Feeding of the Heifer

The heifer is the future milk producer and she has to be given a fair chance to produce well. She must have an average daily gain of at least 500 grams per day in order to reach the optimum size for calving within reasonable time. Unfortunately, many farmers consider heifers to be unproductive and hence they are not properly fed. Lack of feed is often a reality, it is therefore not possible to feed all animals in the herd with high quality feed.

The following advice could be considered as a rule of thumb, bearing in mind that the quantity and quality of feed varies with the season. Furthermore, the condition and growth rate of the heifer should be checked regularly to see that she has the approximate growth rate and if not, adjust her feeding schedule accordingly.

The heifers should be fed green feed of the season of about 4-7 kg DM together with some straw and concentrate or grain per day. If the green feed is leguminous the ration of green feed and concentrate or grain can be reduced and the amount of straw increased. However, it is positive to feed the heifers a small amount of grain or concentrate for making both them and their rumen accustomed to this type of feed, especially partus.

If available, ammonia treated straw could be given along with low quality green feed and concentrate. Silage could be given to heifers, but it is often a very valuable feed saved for milk producing animals. However, a few months before partus the heifer should slowly be introduced to the feed she will have as a milk producing buffalo.

Maximum voluntary intake of the heifer is obtained @ approximately 1 to 1.5 kg dry matter of straw together with 3 kg (DM) of green feed and 1 kg concentrate. Straw fed to appetite is not enough to keep or increase body weight of growing buffaloes. Straw fed to growing stock should preferably be ammoniated and further supplemented with green feed or hay and some kind of concentrate to give the best result.

Feeding of the Dry buffalow

Feeding the dry buffalo concerns preparing for partum and a high milk production. In the last two months of gestation the buffalo has increased requirements for nutrients for fetal growth. Experiments with Murrah buffaloes has shown that the best economical way of feeding dry buffaloes 2 months before calving is at 125 per cent of the recommended level for cattle. By giving the dry buffalo a little more than she needs, her chance to build up the body reserves and to be in good physical condition is improved. After calving the buffalo can be fed at 100 per cent of recommended level for cattle.

MILK PRODUCTION OF THE BUFFALO

The world's milk production from buffaloes was according to FAO (1994) 48 million tons, most of which was produced in Asia (46.5 million tons) by many low producing animals. A great part of the milk production goes unrecorded as the buffalo milk is largely handled by the unorganized sector. For comparison, the world's production of milk from cattle was 459 million tons. In India, Pakistan and Egypt, 65 per cent of the milk produced is from buffaloes.

Lactation and Milk Yield

The onset of lactation is with the birth of the calf. The initial yield is a reliable indicator of the animal's genetic potential. The highest yield is reached after five to six weeks of lactation and maintained for some weeks. Thereafter the yield decreases until the end of lactation. The lactation ends as the dry period starts.

In buffaloes, the highest milk yield is seen in the fourth lactation whereafter it declines. The shape of the lactation curve depends on factors such as feed, management, milking frequency, diseases among others. The optimum lactation length in the Murrah has been reported to be 262 to 295 days.In

Italy it is recommended to keep a lactation length of 270 days in controlled herds. ICAR recommends a lactation length of 305 days as for controlled cattle.

Factors Affecting Lactation and Milk Yield

Lactation and milk yield depend on both genetic and non-genetic factors. The genetic influence is due to species, breed, and individual. Further, it is affected by ability to reproduce, e.g. fertility and thereby calving interval. Improvement on these may be the result of breeding and selection.

The non-genetic factors are management, amount and quality of feed and skill of the farmer to detect heat and illnesses. Factors which are outside the farmer's control such as climate, temperature, humidity etc. also influence lactation and milk yield. Feeding is the most important factor for increasing and sustaining the milk yield. Sufficient amount of energy, protein, minerals and water must be provided in order to achieve maximum yield. See section on Practical feeding of the lactating buffalo.

Calving interval is closely related to lactation length and milk yield. The longer the calving interval, the longer the lactation and the higher the lactation yield. However, total life time yield will be substantially less comparing with a buffalo with short calving intervals. Milking frequency affects both total milk and fat yield. A study using Murrah buffaloes showed that 31 per cent more milk and 26 per cent more butter fat resulted from milking three times per day as compared to twice a day.

Weight of the heifer seems to affect milk yield. Studies on Murrah indicates that the heifers should weigh at least 500 kg at the time of calving in order to reach a maximum milk yield.

Dry Period

The buffalo should be dried off approximately 2 to 3 months before expected calving. The dry period is valuable to the buffalo, she may rest and the udder tissue is repaired.

In a high yielding herd (above 10 kg per day) the buffalo

should be dried off when the daily yield falls below 2.5 kg, even if it is still more than 3 months to expected calving. This goes especially for machine milked herds. An alternative to drying off is to use the buffalo as a foster mother to newly born calves.

One buffalo may serve one newborn calf or two older calves which receive additional feed. Care should be taken to dry her off completely no later than 2 months before calving. In herds which are hand milked and where the yield is low, it is difficult to set a lower limit in kg. Instead, the 2 months limit is recommended.

Composition of Colostrums

During approximately the first three days of lactation the buffalo secretes colostrum. Colostrum is vital for the newborn calf and its composition reflects the calf's need. Colostrum contains the important proteins; the immuno globulins, which are the newborn calf's source of antibodies. The content of iron and copper is markedly higher in the colostrum as compared to normal milk

Alterations of Milk Composition

Milk composition can be altered both before and after the milking. If the change occurs inside the udder it is mostly due to a disease or treatment of the disease by antibiotics or other type of medication. Feeding can alter the normal composition, however, these changes are seldom extreme, but within normal intervals. Season can effect the normal milk composition, although these changes are mostly due to differences in feeding during different seasons.

The fat percentage varies with stage of lactation and with milk yield. A study on Nili-Ravi buffaloes in Pakistan showed that the fat percentage increased steadily from 5.5 per cent in the first month of lactation to 7.5 per cent in the 10th month of lactation.There is a negative correlation between lactation yield and percentage of total solids, fat and protein. However, the total amount of solids, fat and protein is higher in a high yielding buffalo than in a low yielding one.

Feedstuff

A rule of thumb is that roughage increases fat cóntent in milk, whereas concentrate depresses it. This depends on the differences in VFA production in the rumen from the different carbohydrate sources. Digestion of fibre results in a higher proportion of acetic acid and thereby more milkfat. Digestion of concentrate on the other hand, results in a higher proportion of propionic acid which is unfavourable for milkfat synthesis. If too much concentrate is given, fat depression might occur.

Higher energy diets seem to give better coagulation properties of the milk. Long-chain fatty acids increases when the energy concentration in feed is low. Glucosinolates in Brassica spp. are hydrolyzed by the ruminal microbes into thiocyanates, iso- thiocyanates and some other products. Thiocyanate is then excreted in the milk.

High feeding levels with Brassica spp. may therefore lead to unsatisfactory levels of thiocyanate in the milk. Thiocyanate may cause thyroid enlargement in animals as well as humans ingesting it. A common feed stuff of Brassica spp. is mustard fodder and mustard oil cake. Even 15 days after withdrawal of mustard feed, circulatory high levels of thiocyanate exists and is secreted in milk.

Disease and Medication

Mastitis changes the milk composition dramatically. The alterations can sometimes be used as detection of the disease. If antibiotics are used in order to cure for example mastitis, these will be excreted in the milk. Controlling of external parasites with e.g. diazinon affects milk yield as well as composition. The chemical is detected in the milk upto 48 hours after dermal application.

MILKING THE BUFFALO

Buffaloes have been used for milk production for centuries. They have not been subjected to the same upgrading and breeding like cattle of the western world. However, the buffalo is an excellent milk producer, given the correct circumstances. Milking the buffalo is not a difficult task. One should, however, take care not to implement cattle milking techniques directly on the buffalo cow. As described below, the anatomy and physiology of the buffalo udder differs slightly from the bovine one. This has further implications on the milking technique as mentioned later.

The buffalo has an udder similar to the cattle in the gross anatomy. The buffalo has four teats. Extra teats can be found in the similar way as in cattle. The teats vary in shape and size. Generally, they are larger than cattle teats. According to several studies, cylindrical forms of the teats are most common in the Murrah breed. The front teats are, on average, 5.8 cm to 6.4 cm long and their diameter is approximately 2.5 cm to 2.6 cm. Respective figures for the hind teats are 6.9 cm to 7.8 cm and 2.6 to 2.8 cm.

The hind quarters of the udder are slightly larger than the front ones and contain more milk. The approximate ratio is 60:40 (hind:front), as for cattle. It takes a longer time to milk the hind quarters. The anatomy of buffalo teats is slightly different from cattle teats. The epithelium of the streak canal is thicker and more compact in buffaloes than in cattle.

The sphincter muscle around the streak canal is thicker in buffaloes than in cattle. More force is therefore required to open the streak canal. The teat sphincter tonus has been reported to be at least 400 mmHg negative pressure in buffaloes (the tension falls some what after calf suckling and hand milking). This is the cause of buffaloes being "hard milkers".

In cattle, the milk is synthesized in the alveoli and is periodically transferred to the large ducts and cisterns of the mammary gland and the teat. This is not the case in the buffalo, instead, the milk is held in the upper, glandular part of the udder, in the alveoli and small ducts. Between two milkings there is no milk stored in the cistern. Hence, buffaloes have no cisternal milk fraction.

The milk is expelled to the cistern only during actual milk ejection. The same phenomenon is seen in Chinese Yellow cows and Yaks. Because of the absence of cisternal milk between milking, in the teat cisterns, the teats are collapsed and soft before let down. This is contradictory to the bovine cow, where the teats can be very hard and firm due to the presence of milk in the teat cistern.

Physiology of Milking

For a comparison with cattle see booklet on Efficient Milking. Buffaloes are said to be slow and hard milkers because of their slow milk ejection reflex and their hard teat muscle sphincter. The milk ejection reflex appears to be inherited to some extent but it is also a product of the environment. In buffaloes, the let down time averages 2 minutes but may be as long as 10 minutes. The reasons for this are not fully understood.

One reason for the longer let down time of milk for buffaloes is probably the different anatomy of the udder as compared to the dairy cow. In the buffalo, the udder cistern is absent or has a very small volume and therefore there is little or no cisternal milk available. This furthermore leads to no intramammary pressure in the cistern which would otherwise help the milk flow. In cattle, the milk is already stored in the large cistern, and milk is available for extraction immediately after preparation. The high intramammary pressure contributes in pressing out the milk.

The intramammary pressure increases at the onset of milking. It is highest during the peak flow and decreases there after to zero at the end of milking. The pressure is higher in buffaloes during milking than in cattle. The intramammary pressure varies between individuals and milkings. Its' level is not always indicative of a high milk production.

Let down time seems to be negatively correlated to milk yield. Let down time is shorter in early and middle stage of lactation as compared to in late lactation. A faster flow of milk is observed when the yield is higher.If buffaloes are carefully selected for yield and ease to milk, improvement in these characteristics is possible.

Induction of Milk Let Down

Physical stimulation of the teats, either by the calf's

suckling or the milkers hands, excite receptors from which nerve impulses are send to the posterior pituitary gland causing secretion of the hormone oxytocin. The hormone is transported via the blood to the mammary gland. Because both hormones and nerve impulses are involved in the milk ejection reflex, it is called a neurohormonal reflex. Oxytocin stimulates the contraction of the alveoli and small ducts thereby emptying the milk into the larger ducts and the cistern. Hereafter the milk can be evacuated from the udder. See booklet on Efficient Milking.

The contraction of the alveoli may, to some extent, be enhanced by tactile stimuli of the udder (massaging, squeezing) the so called tap reflex. When calves suckle, they butt at the udder in order increase milk secretion. Manual massage of the udder during milking imitates this reflex. Like cattle, buffaloes can get used to different stimuli. It is clear that also in buffaloes, oxytocin release is triggered by visual or audible stimuli, such as the sight of the milker, the noise of the vacuum pump or when entering the milking parlour.

The animal becomes conditioned to let-down milk and has thus developed a conditioned reflex. (An unconditioned reflex is the suckling of the calf.) By letting the animals get accostumed to a strict routine, time of let-down is shortened. In cattle, it has been demonstrated that feeding concentrate during milking improve time of let-down. It has yet to be shown in buffaloes.

Buffaloes are sensitive to changes in the environment. They may withhold the milk if they are uncomfortable with the situation. If the animals are stressed, scared or in pain, the hormone adrenaline is secreted. This hormone causes constriction of the blood vessels, thereby hindering the supply of sufficient amount of oxytocin to the udder. Adrenaline also directly acts on the myoepithelial cells in the alveoli by blocking the oxytocin receptors.

The inhibition if milk let-down will result in the leaving of milk in the secretory parts of the udder. Continuos exposure of stress to the buffaloes will affect the milk production negatively. Change of milker or milking routine, application of wrong milking technique or milking machines in bad conditions are some reasons for the buffaloes to with hold the milk. The actual milking can begin after the let down reflex has been elicited. Whether this is done by hand or machine it is important to use proper routines. The milking should be done as fast as possible without causing stress or pain. The milking should be as complete as possible without excessive stripping. Elevated residual milk in the secretory part of the udder decreases milk secretion and thereby influences the milk yield negatively.

Keeping Good Hygiene

Simple guidelines for keeping good hygiene in the barn or milking parlor:

Dung should be removed both prior to and during milking in order to minimize exposure of the milking equipment to dirt. If the equipment for some reason becomes dirty, it must be cleaned properly before using it again.

- Hands should be clean when milking or handling the milk. Clothes should be clean.
- Use one udder-towel per buffalo, discharge towels in a separate bucket after usage.
- Post-dipping of teats should always be done.
- All containers with milk should have a lid on at all times.
- Milk should not be stored near the dung or feeding place. There are several reasons for this; 1) milk is sensitive to odors and may "pickup" dung or feed odors. 2) Bacteria from dung or feed are more easily transferred to the milk if it is stored nearby. 3) Particles from the dung heap or the feed may contaminate the milk.
- It should not be possible for animals such as dogs, cats and rats to approach the containers.

Pre-milking

Pre-milking is defined as actions to induce milk let-down by cleaning the udder and pre-milk in a strip cup. Cleaning the udder should be done with a lubricated towel (washable textile or disposable paper). Separate towels should be used for each buffalo. The udder should never be splashed with water.

Pre-milking is necessary for various reasons; the most important being preparing the buffalo for actual milking and checking for mastitis or other infections. Pre-milking must be done in a strip cup, never on the floor! The purpose of using a strip cup is to be able to easily observe changes in the milk. Furthermore, the spreading of pathogenic bacteria is limited. Pre-milking is done with dry hands and the fullhand method. The hands should be cleaned between buffaloes during the milking, if necessary.

After Milking

After milking the teats should be disinfected. This reduces, if not completely inhibits, bacterial growth on the teats. The teat canal stays open for a while after milking is completed, thus eliminating the important protection against entry of bacteria. The dip solution will both act as a physical hindrance for bacteria and as a disinfectant. Preferably the teat-dipping-solution should contain some lubricant in order to maintain teat condition and to prevent chapping and sores.

Because the teat canal is open after milking, sometimes for as long as half an hour, the buffaloes should be prevented from lying down. This can be done by giving enough feed to last for a long time after milking.

Special detergents for cleaning of the milking equipment is available and should be used correctly. All buckets, containers and machines used for milking must be cleaned both outwards and inwards immediately after usage. The towels used for cleaning and drying of the udder should be cleaned properly after each milking. They can be stored in a bucket with a lid and clean water containing chloride until the next milking.

Milking Routine

An appropriate milking routine is important for hygienic

and production reasons as well as for creating a comfortable and smooth environment for animals and milkers. It is easier to maintain a good hygiene and to facilitate the adoption by the buffaloes to relief milkers if a consistent milking routine is applied. In dairy cows it has been demonstrated that the practicing of a strict milking routine results in increased milk production.

The routine mentioned below can be followed by both hand and machine milkers in tie-stall barns or where milkings are carried out in flat barns. In the case of hand milking in such barns, points 6 to 9 are omitted. Routine check of the milking machine should be done before each milking session according to the manufacturers recommendation.

- Start by tying (if not already tied) and feeding the buffaloes.
- Remove dung from the floor.
- Wash hands with soap and dry them.
- Clean the teats with special towels and massage them thoroughly.
- Foremilk the buffalo by hand in a strip cup, checking the appearance of the milk.
- Apply the cluster gently. Check tube alignment.
- Check the buffalo every now and then to make sure that she is comfortable with the machine.
- Palpate the udder to check that it feels empty.
- Remove the cluster gently.
- Dip the teats in a suitable disinfectant solution.
- Clean all the equipment in the milking room.

When machine milking, it is important that the milking machine is nearby and ready to be applied to the udder at the right time (after pre-milking). Thus, each buffalo must be cleaned, massaged and pre-milked and then have the machine applied directly.

It must be emphasized that it is not possible to clean all the buffaloes first and then apply the machines to the first buffaloes. The oxytocin release has a short duration (a few minutes). If the machine does not start milking after this time, a whole new procedure must start after half an hour.

Hand Milking

Pre-milking routines are as important when milking buffaloes as when milking cows. For a complete review see Efficient Milking. It is important to use a smooth and comfortable milking technique. The "knuckling" or "stripping" method is used in the wrong belief that it is necessary in order to overcome the resistance in the teat sphincter. These milking methods might cause elongation and damage to the teats. A much more comfortable and appropriate method is the "fullhand" technique. This technique imitates the calf's suckling and is therefore a better stimuli.

Machines for Milking Buffaloes

Since the udder and teats in buffaloes are different compared to cattle, milking machines for cattle have to be modified in order to fit buffaloes. In general, a heavier cluster, a higher operation vacuum and a faster pulsation rate is required. Results from recent studies in India indicate that it might be possible to reduce the cluster weight and the frequency of liner slip by applying an appropriate combination of liner design and cluster weight.

It is not only the total weight of the cluster that is important, but also the distribution of its weight on the udder. Unequal weight distribution can cause uneven milk output. The long milk and vacuum tubes should be aligned and stretched to ensure equal weight distribution of the cluster on the udder. Milking characteristics depend upon vacuum levels and pulsation rates among others. Studies on Egyptian buffaloes revealed that a vacuum of 51 kPa and a pulsation rate of 55 cycles/min led to much longer milking times than a vacuum of 60 kPa and a pulsation rate of 65 cycles/min.

The higher vacuum level, however, caused a significant increase in the somatic cell counts. Highest milk yield within an acceptable time were found when using 56 kPa and 65 cycles/min. In all trials a pulsation ratio of 50:50 was used. Studies in Pakistan indicated that the pulsation rate and ration should be 70 cycles/min and 65:35 respectively for Nili-Ravi buffaloes. In Italy, the majority of farms use the same machines for both buffaloes and cattle. It is a simple "cattle machine" with one vacuum level operating at approximately 40 cm Hg. In India, recent trials have been made with milking with DuovacTM from Alfa Laval Agri.

Successful milking was done with a vacuum level of 55 kPa, 70 cycles/min pulsation rate and pulsation ratio of 65:35 for milk flows above 0.2 kg/min. For milk flows under 0.2 kg/min the respective data where 38 kPa, 48 cycles/min and the same pulsation ratio. The DuovacTM is physiologically correct for the animal since it helps in gently stimulating let-down and is also more gentle to the teats after the peak flow.

In order to obtain all the advantages with machine milking the correct technique must be used. The milkers and buffaloes must be familiar with the machines.

If the buffaloes are scared or feel uncomfortable they will withhold the milk and thereby yield less. This in turn will lead to economic loss for the farmer and eventually he will loose his faith in machine milking.

The concept of machine milking should be introduced slowly and by persons who the buffaloes are used to and feel comfortable with under the supervision of an expert from Alfa Laval Algri.

The procedure of introducing buffaloes to machine milking presented below an recommended by Alfa Laval Agri is applicable for a whole herd where neither animals nor humans are familiar with machine milking. By carefully following the mentioned steps, a successful introduction should be possible.

- *Training of personnel:* Training of milkers should be done by a person from the milking machine company. This person has good knowledge about biology of milking, machine milking as well as with the design, function and maintenance of the milking equipment. The training should include introduction procedures, milking routine, handling of the machine, cleaning and maintenance as well as certain aspects of the day-to-day service of the machine.

- Installation of the milking machine in the barn and any other modification in the barn should be made well in advance of the changing to machine milking.
- It is most appropriate to start with heifers since it is easier to habituate heifers than older buffaloes to machine milking. Older buffaloes may have been hand milked by a certain routine for several lactations and may respond negatively to a change in routine. Heifers on the other hand are not accustomed to any specific routine and are more likely to accept machine milking as well as hand milking. Furthermore their udders and teats are more uniform and not damaged by previous milking. Liner slip and other negative effects of machine milking is therefore less pronounced in heifers. Note that heifers should not be hand milked but directly introduced to the machine. They may get accustomed to the noise of the vacuum pump etc. by participating in the milking routines prior to partus.
- Calm animals that are comfortable with hand milking should be selected. The udders and teats of the animals should be uniform with respect to conformation and size. Buffaloes in heat or unhealthy animals or animals with previous let-down-problems should not be selected.
- Milk the old and selected animals as usual by hand but let the vacuum pump run during milking. This will make the animals accustomed to the noise. Put the pump on before actual milking, but after the buffaloes have been tied up, otherwise the animals may be startled by the sudden noise. Repeat the procedure (usually 2 to 4 times) until all buffaloes are accustomed to the noise. It is better to repeat this procedure once or twice more until all buffaloes are comfortable, than rushing into the next step.
- Bring the milking machines into the barn. Connect them to the airline and place them at each buffalo's place at the same time as hand milking is carried

out. This will allow the buffaloes to get used to the "ticking" sound of the pulsator. It will give them a chance to look at the machines and smell them and may be even taste them. Make sure though, that they do not chew on them! Move the machines to the next buffalo in order to milked. This makes the buffaloes used to machines being moved around. The procedure should be repeated (usually 2 to 4 times) until all the animals have accepted the presence of the machines.

At this stage, presumably all buffaloes will be well accustomed to the new routine. If some buffaloes are still showing signs of nervousness or stress, it is recommended to repeat the above mentioned steps until the animals are calm. Buffaloes that after this procedure have not accepted being milked by machines should be returned to hand milking. One or two frightened or uncomfortable buffaloes might cause major disturbances in the whole herd.

Consistency with respect to milking routine including pre-milking preparation should be applied from the beginning of the introduction period. The regular milker should carry out the machine milking during the introduction period. When the cluster is firmly attached to the udder, the milker should stay with the buffalo to see that she is comfortable. Soft talking and brushing and scratching are the best ways to calm an animal. These first sessions of machine milkings usually require longer time than the following. However, this time is well worth spending to assure forward calm and easy-milking buffaloes.

MASTITIS

Mastitis, inflammation of the mammary gland, is a common disease in dairy animals. The disease causes great economic losses both for farmers and for dairies. A recent study in India revealed that sub clinical mastitis causes an annual loss of 604.000 rupees in cows and 483.000 in buffaloes. Respective figures for clinical mastitis is 285.000 and 235.000 rupees. Total loss caused by mastitis in buffaloes is calculated to 717.000 rupees in buffaloes.

Mastitis may be caused by several factors. Most important and most common is bacterial infection. Good hygiene practice is the most efficient way of preventing the disease from developing and spreading. Mastitis may also be caused by trauma such as injuries on the udder or the teat. Sores are a perfect way of entry for bacteria.

The most common bacteria causing mastitis in buffaloes are Staphylococcus (Staph. epidermis and Staph. Aureus), Streptococcus (Str. dysgalactia and agalactia) and Coryonebacterium spp. This is not very different from the incidence of respective bacteria in cattle mastitis. There is, however, a difference in bacteriology of the mastitis due to the kind or farm the buffaloes come from. On rational, modern farms, the most common bacteria causing mastitis is often Staph. aureus. On traditional farms, Streptococcus faecalis, Escherichia coli and Clostridium perfringens are the most prevalent.

An Italian study reported that mastitis was more frequent on modern farms and that this was caused by high production, causing heavy stress on the udder, and trauma to the teats caused by milking machine. The bacteria were a mere secondary infection. On the other hand, on traditional farms, mastitis was less frequent but was caused by lack of even the most simple hygienic routines. This is shown by the bacteria causing mastitis in traditional farms, they are purely fecal and soil bacteria.

This is confirmed by a recent study in Italy where buffaloes where randomly tested for somatic cell count and total bacteria count together with CMT. 66 per cent of the buffaloes showed an abnormal high number of SCC in the milk. These buffaloes where kept in a traditional Italian loose house system, which indicates that the hygieneic standards could be improved. Mastitis seems to be more frequent in animals with high milk yield, both regarding individuals, herds, breeds and species.

This may have to do with the higher stress that the udder is exposed to when yielding more milk. It is quite clear however, that buffaloes are less susceptible to mastitis than cattle. There might be both anatomical and physiological reasons for this. A recent Indian study has compiled data on incidence of mastitis in cows as well as in buffaloes,

Mastitis can be clinical and sub-clinical. There is an important difference between these two. Sub-clinical mastitis may not even show. The observant milker may see slight changes in the milk like the appearance of flakes, when fore milking in the strip cup. Sub-clinical mastitis shows in the CMT. Acute mastitis is detected very easily. The udder is sore, swollen, hot and red. The buffalo is in pain when the inflamed quarter is touched.

An inflamed quarter should be milked by hand very carefully, not forcing the milk out. This may be quite difficult, since the milk is thick (more like jelly) and may contain blood. The milk should not come into contact with any containers used for milking, nor animals or the floor. It should be wasted. The milker should carefully wash his hands before touching any other quarter, animal or equipment. These rules can not be over emphasized. Never milk an inflamed quarter with a machine!

Buffaloes have a powerful defence against mastitis due to the anatomy of the teat. Starting with the teat skin, the buffalo teat skin is less sensitive than cow teats to chapping and sores. Inside the streak canal, the epithelium is thicker and more compact than in cattle. This gives extra resistance against penetration of bacteria through the epithelium. Furthermore, the keratin layer of the streak canal is thicker. The importance of the keratin layer is that it contains bactericidal and bacteristatic lipids and cationic proteins.

The cationic proteins are inhibitory to the growth of Streptococcus agalactica and Staphylococcus aureus. The sphincter of the streak canal is, as mentioned before, tighter than in cattle. It is also supplied with more nerve fibers and a richer blood vessel system, than in cattle. This will help maintaining a tight closure of the duct thus limiting entry of bacteria in to the mammary gland.

When the udder gets infected or inflamed, the natural defence system goes into action to eliminate the infection or inflammation. Blood leukocytes, especially the phagocytes, migrate through the alveolar epithelium to the milk in order to remove the invading pathogens. Neutrophils are the most active leukocytes in this process. Lymphocytes and macrophages are also important in the udder defence. Neutrophils, lymphocytes and macrophages together with epithelial cells exists in normal milk.

In buffalo milk, several studies have revealed that the amount of neutrophils in total somatic cells (SCC) are as much as 22-88 per cent with an average of 56 per cent. Lymphocytes are in the order of 10-54 per cent (mean 28 per cent). The occurrence of macrophages in buffalo milk is less than in cattle milk (8 per cent vs. 30 per cent). This massive attack by neutrophils is a powerful defence by the udder against invading pathogens.

Cell counts in milk from healthy buffaloes varies between 50.000 and 375.000 per ml. This is comparable to cattle milk and the difference therefore lies in the differential cell count as described above. Studies indicate that the concentration and functional efficiency of phagocytes are superior in buffaloes compared to cattle. The disease is cured with antibiotics. Treating buffaloes in the dry period with antibiotics in order to prevent the disease has shown to be very effective.

However, this can not be advisable since bacteria are known to develop resistance. Instead good methods for preventing the disease should be practiced. With training to detect mastitis during the early phase, spread of the disease can be prevented.

Mastitic Milk

Acute mastitis is easily detected by looking at the milk or at the udder. The milk is more or less jelly-like and contains flakes. This change in appearance is mostly due to an increase in cell count and bacterial count. Very often there is blood in the milk. Somatic cell count is drastically increased in mastitic milk. The salt (NaCl) concentration is higher (as much as 33 per cent) and potassium concentration is lower in mastitic milk. Increases in magnesium and calcium are also detectable. The lactose content is much lower than in normal milk, it can be reduced by 16 per cent. The fat concentration can be reduced by 45 per cent in some cases. Mastitic milk should always be discarded, never delivered to the dairies and not given to the calves.

Machine milking has both been praised as the solution to mastitis problems and been cursed as the cause of mastitis. None of these extremes are completely true but in some cases milking with machines can aid in developing mastitis or facilitating its spreading. As stated previously, incorrect use of milking machines or milking with machines in poor condition may cause trauma to the teats.

This in turn may lead to injuries like sores or chapping. The sores are readily invaded by pathogenic organisms and the disease is a fact. If a buffalo already has got an infected quarter, machines may aid in transmitting pathogens to the other quarters or to another buffalo. A fluctuating vacuum may cause milk to be pressed into the teat again, thus invading the teat with pathogens.

The machines themselves may also be a source for pathogens. Old liners and rubbers are easily cracked, in these cracks micro-organisms are less susceptible to washing and detergents and may survive the cleaning. All these factors may easily be eliminated by a good hygienic practice as mentioned above and by keeping the equipment in good condition.

A good hygiene and quality can only be maintained if care is taken when handling the milk. Milk should be stored in containers solely used for this purpose. A lid which fits tightly prevents dirt as well as insects to enter the container. The containers must be thoroughly cleansed after usage. Milk containers should be handled with care, milk is sensitive to stirring and shaking as this may damage the fat globules, leading to spoiled milk.

COOLING

The effect of cooling can not be over emphasized. It is the best means to preserve the quality of milk and to prevent bacteria from multiplying. Cooling of milk does not necessary require expensive cooling equipment. Some simple and cheap methods are listed below. In order to obtain the best results with these methods, the container should be of metal for fast heat exchange.

Shade and draught provide some cooling to the fresh milk. Covering the container with a wet cloth is a successful way of obtaining additional cooling from water evaporation. This is particularly useful in dry climates. Air cooling is most effective at night. Evening milk may be stored without severe problems until next morning if the air temperature is 10°C, or below.

The milk container is put in the coldest water available. Preferably a metal basin or earthen pit with running water, so that the water never warms up. A stream functions equally well. For this type of cooling the milk container should not be heavier than that it is possible to lift for one man.

A slightly more sophisticated way of cooling with water is by having a metal basin with double walls. The milk is poured into the basin and heat is exchanged with the water running in the double wall. This requires some kind of stirring and a large lid. For water cooling to be efficient, the temperature of the water should not exceed 20°C. It also requires a rich supply of clean water. The water used for cooling may be given to the buffaloes after it has served its purpose. In this way, water is saved.

It is quite effective but expensive. It works by putting blocks of ice around the milk container. However, even though the ice is colder than water, it may not work as well due to bad contact between the surfaces. A metal box containing ice can be inserted into the milk. This requires strict hygiene and clean boxes. It is not advisable to put ice into the milk. Firstly the milk becomes diluted and, secondly, if the water is not perfectly clean, it will add bacteria to the milk.

If ice is readily available and not to expensive it can be combined with water cooling, thus chilling the water further.

Mechanical cooling can be more or less expensive. If the farmer has a household refrigerator, this can be used for cooling the milk. How large a quantity of milk depends on the size of the refrigerator. Sophisticated coolers for chilling larger quantities of milk quickly are available from many agricultural companies. Air, water and ice cooling can be used in combination with mechanical cooling. By first cooling the milk in air, water or ice, some energy for further mechanical cooling is saved. Buffalo milk is mainly produced in the rural areas by a multitude of small farmers.

In developing countries, high temperatures and long transportation times in unsanitary containers contribute to rapid increase of bacteria and thereby a large amount of the milk is spoiled before it reaches the dairy plant to be processed. Poor infrastructure discourages farmers to deliver the milk themselves to the dairy plant. Instead they deliver it to collection centres which may be organized by the dairy plant or by the farmers themselves as a cooperative or by businessmen or organizations.

Most collection centres are merely a simple shed where milk is weighed and perhaps tested for fat, then transported to the dairy plant on a truck twice a day. More modern collection centres may have facilities to cool the milk or even a cooling tank and it is sufficient to transport the milk to the dairy once a day.

Decentralized dairy plants which can be reached from many farms within two hours is another solution to minimize spoilage of milk. Transportation of the milk should preferably be done in large containers since a large quantity of milk heats up more slowly a small quantity. Increases in temperature during the transportation should be avoided as much as possible.

If cooling of the milk is impossible, preservatives can be used to retain milk quality until it reaches the dairy. It must be emphasized that a preservative does nothing but preserve the milk, it can not in any way improve the quality of the milk. An available preservative is lactoperoxidase/ hydrogen peroxide/ thiocyanate and the method is commonly called the LP-system or MIPS. It is a safe method of preserving milk if used correctly and it does not affect the quality of the milk negatively. For full description of the system contact Alfa Laval Agri.

Quality Control

The aim of quality control is to assure that the milk purchased from the farmers has a good hygienic standard and a normal composition. A very easy and simple quality control can be done at farm level or at the collection centre by trained personnel. There are simple check points that should be looked at in order to determine quality.

- Overall hygiene in the milking area
- Cleanliness of the milk containers
- Milking routines
- Cooling facilities
- Cleaning procedure

These points should be checked regularly at the farm. The staff conducting this should do so without prior notice to the farmer. It is the farmers' responsibility to always keep clean and have good milking routines. Any one should be able to check on his routines at any time and find them satisfactory. If the farmer does not have satisfactory cleaning and cleanliness, he should receive advice from the staff as to how he can improve his conditions.

REPRODUCTION

The water buffalo has a reputation for being a sluggish breeder, but the average animal is so poorly fed that it's reproductive performance is unrepresentative of it's capabilities. Without reasonable nutrition the animals cannot reach puberty as early in life or reproduce as regularly as their physiology or genetic capabilities would normally allow.

With good management, adequately nourished buffaloes can reach puberty at about the same age as cattle, as early as 18 months of age in buffalo bulls. In northern Australia, Swamp females have conceived at 16 months of age. In the herd at Punjab Agricultural University in Ludiana, India, 11 River buffalo heifers showed estrus at ages less than 18.5 months and a few came into heat when less than 15 months old.

The water buffalo also can calve at an age comparable to that of cattle. At the Ain Shams University in Egypt a well fed

Egyptian buffalo herd of several hundred animals has an average age at first calving of 27 months, 22 days. Because of uncertainties, El Ashry and his colleagues believe that the body weight is a better indicator of sexual preparedness than age. These researchers at Ain Shamus University recommended mating heifers when they weigh 365 kg no matter what their age. Research at Punjub Agricultural University shows that heifers can be bred when they weigh over 270 kg and manifest estrus. Most animals in the Punjab Agricultural University River buffalo herd calved before 35 months, one at 28.3 months.

In one Venezuelan herd almost all heifers 20-24 months old were pregnant; virtually all calved before age 38 months, most by 30 months, and one at age 23 months. In trials in Queensland, Australia and in Papua New Guinea it was noticed that female buffaloes (Swamp breed) came into estrus even while they were losing weight because of adequate nutrition, whereas cattle did not.

Under these stressful conditions the buffalo calves also reached sexual maturity earlier and the buffaloes had a higher calving percentage and a shorter calving interval because they came back into estrus more quickly than cattle. The age at first calving of more than 60 nutritionally poor buffaloes was 38 months in one herd and 45 months for Brahman cross cattle.

Similar observations have been made in Florida. Trinidad, the Brazilian Amazon, Venezuela, and elsewhere. Although these are exceptions to the normal observations in Asia, where buffaloes seem to breed more slowly than cattle, they do demonstrate the buffalo's potential for improved breeding.

Unclean surroundings, poor nutrition, and poor management, causes a great number of early embryonic deaths and a high death rate among the calves; this also contributes to the buffalo's often low reproductive rate.

Female Reproduction

Estrus

Oestrus, estrus or heat is a specific period of reproductive function when the female becomes receptive. Estrus in buffaloes is manifested by changes in the reproductive system and in behaviour. It usually lasts about 24 hours, but duration varies and may range from 11 to 72 hours. It occurs on an average of 21 day cycles. Determination of when a buffalo cow is in estrus is difficult because often the animal shows few external signs of "heat". This increases the chances of missing a cycle, especially for artificial insemination.

The intensity of estrus behaviour in Egyptian and Indian buffaloes has been found to be much less than cows. The usual weak symptoms of estrus in the normal breeding season (October to February in Asia and India) become still weaker during the hot months of summer. Unlike most of the buffalo breeds of tropical and temperate regions, the symptoms of estrus in Philippine buffaloes have been reported to be even more pronounced than cattle.

The problems of estrus detection in Swamp buffalo of Thailand has been described as one of the main constraints of the breeding programme.

Diurnal patterns of estrus behaviour have been observed in most buffaloes. The Swamp usually breed at night. In about 855 of Egyptian and Indian buffaloes signs of estrus have been recorded between 6 pm and 6 am. However during monsoon, estrus often commences in the afternoon hours.

In the Phillipines the management concept of night corrals has been used to increase reproductive performance. Due to the high incidence of silent heat large numbers of buffaloes are left unbred. In Egyptian buffaloes 86 per cent silent heat has been reported. In Indian buffaloes, one study showed only 15 per cent silent heat. Work on estrus synchronisation using has been done in New Zealand.

Estrus Detection

Frequent urination is the most reliable symptom of estrus. The animals urinate small quantities every 4-6 minutes in some cases. Mucus vaginal discharge in quietly sitting animals can also be observed. Many buffaloes show clear or transparent cervical mucus at the onset of estrus which becomes cloudy and turbid to dirty translucent with the advancement of the estrus. For the detection of estrus in buffaloes the application of a combination of aids has been suggested.

- A vasectomized or teaser buffalo bull should be paraded in the morning and in the evening in the area where open buffaloes are kept. Interest by the bull or the female buffalo mounting upon the bull or showing affinity for the bull should be indicate heat. This procedure can be increased to three time a day during the peak breeding seasons. In many areas, vasectomized bulls are not available and an intact animal that has been suitably trained and accustomed to control can be used. This method is most suitable in operations where the cows are confined in station alleys. The ability, observation skills, and training of the bull handler are extremely important in this method.
- Breedable open buffaloes should be regularity checked at 3-4 hour intervals for vaginal discharge. Mucus discharge from the vagina flows as a string from the vulva of animals in heat. The thick stringy appearance is characteristic. The inner side of the tail should be examined for vaginal discharge.
- Cervical mucus should be collected and spread over a clean microscopic slide and left for drying at room temperature. Typical fern pattern crystallization indicates estrus.
- Suspect animals should be examined through rectal palpation for uterus tone and the presence of mature follicles on the ovary.
- Under freestall or pasture conditions a vasectomized bull with a marker apparatus may be left loose with the cows. Tailhead chalk, paint or other marking devices can also be useful to detect "riding"...even if a vasectomized bull is not available.
- In hot weather both female and males should be protected from direct solar radiation and heat stress. Some studies have shown the value of water spray

cooling and sprinkling in intensifying the signs and extending the duration of estrus.

Estrus Duration

In young Murrah buffaloes in India average estrus period has been observed to be 29 (24-72) hours. Other studies have shown variations according to location, breed and season...24 hrs in the Philippines...12-36 hrs in Egypt...24-36 hrs in Bulgaria and 19.5 (with a range of 3 to 69 hrs. in Pakistan. The duration of estrus is usually slightly longer...and more regular in aged than in young buffaloes. An estrus duration of about 24 hours is usually used for practical purposes. Similar to other bovines, the estrus cycle in buffaloes can be approximately divided into phases...

Proestrus

The ovary is more active. FSH hormone stimulates the growth of follicles. This proestrus period of the cycle is also called the follicular phase or..due to the rising levels of estrogen it is called the estrogenic phase. The increased secretion of estrogen from growing follicles increases blood supply and growth of tubular genitalia. Various degrees of swelling of the vulva due to congestion may be seen and mucus secretion may start. The duration of proestrus may be 2-3 days.

Estrus

Characterized by the typical breeding behaviour of females. The animal becomes restless and urinates frequently. there is stringy clear mucus discharge from the vagina with marked edema of internal and external genitalia. During this period females are ready for mating and ovulation usually takes place about 5-24 hours after the cessation of estrus signs. In the latter part of estrus secretion of LH increases and that of FSH decreases. This changed pattern of hormone secretion causes ovulation and then formation of corpus luteum (CL) in the ovary.

Metaestrus

This phase is 3-4 days. During this period there is a sharp

decline in the levels of estrogen and early development takes place. The vulva shrinks to the original form, tubular genitalia return to normal size and the flow of mucus becomes cloudy, thinner and gradually stops.

Dioestrus

During this period the CL remains functional with high levels of progesterone. In cases of conception the CL remains throughout the gestation period for the normal maintenance of pregnancy. When there is no successful fertilization of ovum the dioestrus phase lasts from 10 to 20 days or sometimes longer.

Gestational Estrus

The condition of gestational estrus or heat signs after a successful breeding has been observed in 6-18 per cent of buffaloes (R). Animals which return to heat after service should always be examined for ovarian structure before rebreeding and if follicular status is vague, AI service should be placed outside the cervix rather than thru it into the uterine horn.

One important limiting factor influencing the productivity of buffaloes is the seasonality of breeding. This may be due to anoestrus or silent estrus during the non breeding season. Temperature, humidity, light periods and nutrition have all been mentioned as causes of this seasonality.

Postpartum Estrus

The appearance of estrus signs following parturition is known as post partum estrus. The literature shows ranges of from 10 to 400 days. Again environment, nutrition and heat detection has significant influence on the length of this period. 30-60 days is considered an average return time. In Punjab, India, River buffaloes have been observed to come into estrus as early as 40 days after calving.

Male Reproduction

In general the buffalo bull is very similar to other bovines. The volume of buffalo semen ranges from 1.5 to 5.0 ml per ejaculate and semen quality is influenced by many factors. Most bulls are put into service between 18 and 24 months although environment, management and nutrition significantly influence their sexual activity.

Young bulls less than 24 months, average volume (1.91 ml), initial mortality (22.8 per cent), count of live spermatozoa (46.4 per cent) and density of spermatozoa (107.14x10(6) per ml) indicate the poor quality of semen. This improved significantly in bulls of 2-8 years. Training of buffalo bulls for semen collection usually starts at 20-24 months.

Loss of potency has been observed by 6-7 years but many bulls remain fertile beyond 9 years however the largest period of usefulness is between 3 and 7 years.A good bull can serve about 100 buffalo cows per year in natural service. In many parts of the world artificial insemination is practiced, however much of the population depends upon natural service by free living buffalo bulls of improved breed (mostly Murrah), stray nondescript bulls or entire working buffalo males. Distance of AI centres, frequent closure, and awkward times of estrus are the usual problems. Usually one buffalo bull operates in 2-4 villages having 200-300 breedable females in most parts of Nepal and India. These bulls serve a good number of animals during their active life. Some bulls are seen covering cows even after 10 years although with more enthuasism than effect.

In theory, the quantity and quality of semen collected successfully up to an average 8.75 ejaculates daily is almost identical. The calculated daily spermatozoa production capacity of bulls has been found to be 2.3-2.5 billion. However, in practice this is not possible due to decreased libido and natural endurance problems. Thus the use of buffalo bulls for natural breeding or semen collection should be organized in a systematic manner for optimum utilization.

Buffalo bulls should probably be used not more than 75 times a year....however in most areas about 75 per cent of the services are required during 4 months of the peak breeding season. Breeding bulls should be used 3 times per week during the peak breedng season. Each mating should comprise two services with about a 15 minute interval.

Artificial Insemination

This technique for breeding buffaloes can be used for progeny improvement programmes, optimum usage of good breeding bulls and ease of transportation to remote locations. AI was started in the early forties at Allahabad Agricultural Institute in India, and the first buffalo calf was born on 21 August, 1943.Since the semen of each ejaculate is multiplied through the use of suitable extenders for the breeding of larger numbers of females it is essential to use semen of high quality. This increases the probability of high conception and the introduction of desired traits in the progeny.

Semen Characteristics

In practice maximum rate of collection is on alternate days during the peak breeding season and twice weekly during the rest of the year.

For semen evaluation the determination of initial or mass motility of undiluted semen is an important quick test. The initial motility is either judged by the movements and waves (swirls) in a drop of semen under the microscope on a 0 to 5 scale (sometimes 0 to 10) or by counting the total and non-motile spermatozoa with the help of a hemocytometer. The former gives a rough estimate and the later provides actual percentages of motile sperm in the semen. The average mass motility of Murrah semen has been reported to be 3 to 4. Good cooling arrangements significantly improve the motility.

Morphology

A normal sperm of the buffalo is constituted of 3 distinct parts...head, mid piece and tail. It resembles a balloon with an attached string or a tadpole. The head of the buffalo spermatozoan is more rectangular than that of cattle. Head length, breadth, and shape can be affected by extenders season, number of ejaculates and handling of the ejaculate.

This is determined by counting the percentage of motile sperm in semen diluted to contain about 20 million sperm per ml. The percentage of motility in fresh diluted semen of nondescript buffalo bulls was 67, which gradually decreased after storage at 4-6C. The motility was 40 after 5 days and 30 after 8 days of storage in egg yolk glucose bicarbonate extender. A wide variation in motility, from 45 per cent to 85 per cent has been reported for the buffalo bull In the same sample 65 per cent in fresh whole semen, 75 per cent in fresh diluted semen and 62 per cent in diluted semen frozen in ministraws and then thawed was observed.

The percentage of live and dead sperm is determined by counting of slides prepared by a differential staining technique. The nigrosine eosin stain is widely used for differential staining of buffalo spermatozoa. A wide variation in the ratio of live and dead sperm of buffalo semen has been found. Again age, breed, frequency of collection, season, extender, temperature and handling all influence the percentage. Averages of 75 per cent to 85 per cent live in fresh collections are expected but 40 per cent is commonly seen.

Abnormal Sperm

A large variety of abnormalities in the structure of sperms have been reported. The ratio of normal and abnormal is used as a parameter for the determination of semen quality. 2 per cent to 20 per cent is seen with about 6 per cent being average. The development of efficient extenders for the preservation of live spermatozoa and their fertility for extended time requires knowledge of detailed chemical composition of spermatozoa and seminal plasma.

A significantly lower initial content of fructose in the semen of the buffalo was observed. However, later work has indicated that this is probably a handling defect. Chloride content is higher and citric acid lower. Several specialized extenders for buffalo semen have been developed.

The life span of unprocessed spermatozoa in whole warm semen is limited to a few hours The high temperature has been found unsuitable and the rate of deterioration is rapid due to increased metabolic processes. Cooling can extend this life for several days... however if the temperature becomes too low crystallization of water occurs within the cells and they can be damaged. Therefore for freezing semen needs to be extended in a suitable medium which is little affected by the freezing process. Glycerol has been found to protect the sperm considerably from the freezing process. Deep freezing of buffalo semen was started in India in 1955. Limited research has been done on freezing buffalo semen and even after 50 years of research it is not in wide use nor of equal quality as cattle semen. About 80 per cent recovery of motile spermatozoa on thawing of deep frozen buffalo semen in egg yolk glycine extender has been reported.

Pregnancy percentages from the insemination of thawed semen preserved deep frozen for several months have been reported at 40 per cent to 70 per cent. Reasonable quality deep frozen semen is now commercially available in some areas and it's use is spreading. Overall conception rates of 70-80 percent are reported. It is estimated that some 100,000 buffaloes are now being artificially inseminated.

Pregnancy

The pregnancy is an important reproductive function... and should be the objective of every reproductive programme. Unfortunately focus is sometimes lost and the breeding or insemination numbers are stressed and used to evaluate livestock development programmes. In buffaloes, development of the fetus occurs in the uterine cornua and involvement of the right cornua is much more common than the left. Corpora lutea are almost always present in the ovary of the same side. Recto-vaginal palpation of the gravid uterus is the most common method for diagnosis of pregnancy in both buffaloes and cows.

Diagnosis of pregnancy in the buffalo before 2-3 months of gestation is difficult, especially for those with little experience and practice. At many AI centres the non return of inseminated animals is considered as a measure of pregnancy which may be true due to large numbers of available entire males. Recently progesterone levels in blood, plasma or serum, and milk has been used for diagnosis at early stages of gestation. Hopefully, the use of these techniques will provide improved evaluation of buffalo reproductive programmes.

In many areas, calving is seasonal. This seems to be largely due to changes in nutrition. It may also be caused by heat stress, in either males or females, which results in a low breeding rate during the hot seasons. However, when buffalo cows are well fed and cooled, they come into estrus and will breed in any season.

A wide variation in the conception rate of buffaloes has been reported by different observers. Most values are based on non return rates of the inseminated buffaloes for reinsemination. Rates of 50-60 per cent are average for natural service and half that for most evaluated AI field services. The colour and consistency of cervical mucus has a significant influence on the conception rates.

When mucus changes from transparent to turbid and the crystallization pattern is normal fern like, the conception rate is highest. Many natural matings take place at night and are therefore unobserved. In one set of pregnancy diagnoses in northern Australia, the buffalo's conception rate (81 per cent) was higher than that of the Brahman crossbreeds (70 per cent) they were with.

The length of time required to carry the result of conception to it's full term under normal physiological environment is known as gestation period.The water buffalo's gestation period is about one month longer and is more variable than that of cattle. Whereas cattle give birth after about 280 days(Angus, 279,Holstein, 279-280, Brown Swiss,286), buffaloes take 300-334 days (average 310) or roughly 10 months and 10 days.

In Egypt, the average period according to a study of 424 gestations, is 316+/- 8 days. The development of the fetus in buffaloes is affected by many factors such as breed, type, parity, season, nutritional status, sex of calf and geographical location). Wide variation in the gestation period of River(300-315 days) and Swamp (320-340 days) buffalo has been observed).

Dilation of the cervix, expulsion of the fetus, and detachment of the placenta are all similar to other bovines. Involution of the uterus averages about 30-50 days. The definition of pregnancy rate is: detection of estrus (per cent) times conception rate (per cent). The detection of estrus can be defined as the number of cows in estrus per 21 days divided by number of cows in the breeding group. Pregnancy rate includes all cows in the breeding group whether or not insemination has occurred. It is the best reproductive managment tool available for buffalo but not widely used.

Calving Interval

The interval between the subsequent calvings is known as calving interval or intercalving period. It is a significant reproductive trait for the assessment of the life time production potential of buffaloes. Similar to other reproductive traits the calving interval is also widely variable.

Range of 334-580 days with mean of about 465 days in River buffaloes and 350-800 days with a 553 mean in the Swamp. Only under uncommon circumstances can a buffalo cow produce a calf each year. In one herd of 800 cows in Venezuela the average female buffalo over 4 produces 2 calves every 3 years.

In response to a recent questionnaire, the majority of Indonesian farmers estimated that the calving rate was between 3 and 5 calves in 5 years. A few claimed a calf a year, some only 1 or 2 calves in 5 years. In Florida it has been noted that some buffalo cows having just calved became pregnant more quickly than cattle, so that a calf may indeed be produced each year.

Calving intervals of 14-15 months have been reported in Egypt and Venezuela. Regular yearly breeding has been noted also in northern Australia. Preliminary results in northern Australia indicate that weaning can be carried out as late as 12 months of age without any effect on conception times of the buffalo dam.

Service Period

The interval between calving and conception is known service period. The shorter the service period the longer would be productive life. 100 to 150 days is reported.

Dry Period

The interval between the end of lactation and subsequent calving is called dry period. A minimum dry period of 60 days has been suggested as resting period which helps in rebuilding of body reserves and mammary tissue. Dry periods of 0 to 250 days have been reported with about 150 days average.

Reproductive Failures

Anestrus Anatomical, hereditary, functional and nutritional conditions either singly or in combination produce anestrus in buffaloes. It is highest during the hot months and has characterized the buffalo as a seasonal breeder. Small, hard inactive ovaries are the rule rather than the exception in most buffalo of the world.

Perhaps as newer management methods are developed we will see more information and research on this important constraint to buffalo reproduction. The major cause of infertility in Asian buffaloes is subactive ovaries. Poor feeding, nutritional deficiencies and parasites are the main cause of ovarian inactivity and excessive follicular atresia with the failure of maturation and ovulation.

Ovary Pathology

Hypojunctions, cysts, persistent CL and encapsulation of ovaries are common observations in buffalo. One should consider that many of these reports are from the observation of collected genitalia in slaughter facilities.... from old animals at the end of their useful life.

Tubular Genitalia Salpingitis has been reported as much higher in buffalo than cattle(R). Cervicitis, metritis, pyometra and vaginitis have all been observed but again many of these reports are from slaughter animals. A high number of iatrogenic tubular genital problems occur in AI programmes because of rough handling and poor technique.

Chapter 7

Animal Products

Dairy products are generally defined as foodstuffs produced from milk. They are usually high-energy-yielding food products. A production plant for such processing is called a dairy or a dairy factory. Raw milk for processing generally comes from cows, but occasionally from other mammals such as goats, sheep, water buffalo, yaks, or horses. Dairy products are commonly found in European, Middle Eastern and Indian cuisine, whereas they are almost unknown in East Asian cuisine.

A dairy is a facility for the extraction and processing of animal milk—mostly from goats or cows, but also from buffalo, sheep, camels —for human consumption. As an adjective, the word *dairy* describes milk-based products and processes, dairy cattle, dairy goat. A dairy farm produces milk and a dairy factory processes it into a variety of dairy products.

In New Zealand English a *dairy* means a corner shop, milk bar or Superette and *dairy factory* is the term for what is elsewhere a *dairy*. In the UK a *dairy* is a processing facility that turns milk into a range of products. In the U.S. a *dairy* can be the storage and processing facility for milk, the facility that processes and distributes the milk or the store that sells milk, butter, cheese and suchlike.

Milk-producing animals have been domesticated for thousands of years. Initially they were part of the subsistence farming that nomads engaged in. As the community moved about the country so did their animals accompany them. Protecting and feeding the animals were a big part of the symbiotic relationship between the animal and the herder. In the more recent past, people in agricultural societies owned dairy animals that they milked for domestic or local (village) consumption, a typical example of a cottage industry.

The animals might serve multiple purposes. In this case the animals were normally milked by hand and the herd size was quite small so that all of the animals could be milked in less than an hour—about 10 per milker.

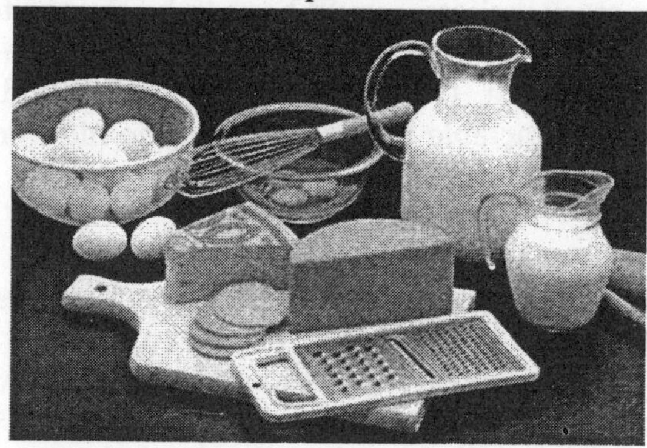

Fig. Dairy Products

With industrialisation and urbanisation the supply of milk became a commercial industry with specialised breeds of cow being developed for dairy, as distinct from beef or draught animals. Initially more people were employed as milkers but it soon turned to mechanisation with machines designed to do the milking. Historically, the milking and the processing took place close together in space and time: on a dairy farm. People milked the animals by hand; on farms where only small numbers are kept hand-milking may still be practiced.

Hand-milking is accomplished by grasping the teats (often pronounced *tit* or *tits*) in the hand and expressing milk either by squeezing the fingers progressively, from the udder end to the tip, or by squeezing the teat between thumb and index finger then moving the hand downward from udder towards the end of the teat. The action of the hand or fingers is designed to close off the milk duct at the udder (upper) end and, by the movement of the fingers, close the duct progressively to the tip to express the trapped milk. Each half or quarter of the udder is emptied one milk-duct capacity at a time.

The *stripping* action is repeated, using both hands for speed. Both methods result in the milk that was trapped in the milk duct being squirted out the end into a bucket that is supported between the knees (or rests on the ground) of the milker, who usually sits on a low stool. Traditionally the cow, or cows, would stand in the field or paddock while being milked.

Young stock, heifers, would have to be trained to remain still to be milked. In many countries the cows were tethered to a post and milked. The problem with this method is that it relies on quiet, tractable beasts, because the hind end of the cow is not restrained.

Processing

When it became necessary to milk larger numbers of cows, the cows would be brought to a shed or barn that was set up with bails (stalls) where the cows could be confined while they were milked. One person could milk more cows this way, as many as 20 for a skilled worker. But having cows standing about in the yard and shed waiting to be milked is not good for the cow, as she needs as much time in the paddock grazing as is possible.

It is usual to restrict the twice-daily milking to a maximum of an hour and a half each time. It makes no difference whether one milks 10 or 1000 cows, the milking time should not exceed a total of about three hours each day for any cow.

As herd sizes increased there was more need to have efficient milking machines, sheds, milk-storage facilities (vats), bulk-milk transport and shed cleaning capabilities and the means of getting cows from paddock to shed and back. Farmers found that cows would abandon their grazing area and walk towards the milking area when the time came for milking. This is not surprising as, in the flush of the milking season, cows presumably get very uncomfortable with udders engorged with milk, and the place of relief for them is the milking shed.

As herd numbers increased so did the problems of animal health. In New Zealand two approaches to this problem have been used. The first was improved veterinary medicines (and the government regulation of the medicines) that the farmer could use. The other was the creation of *veterinary clubs* where groups of farmers would employ a veterinarian (vet) full-time and share those services throughout the year.

It was in the vet's interest to keep the animals healthy and reduce the number of calls from farmers, rather than to ensure that the farmer needed to call for service and pay regularly.

Most dairy farmers milk their cows with absolute regularity at a minimum of twice a day, with some high-producing herds milking up to four times a day to lessen the weight of large volumes of milk in the udder of the cow. This daily milking routine goes on for about 300 to 320 days per year that the cow stays in milk. Some small herds are milked once a day for about the last 20 days of the production cycle but this is not usual for large herds.

If a cow is left unmilked just once she is likely to reduce milk-production almost immediately and the rest of the season may see her *dried off* (giving no milk) and still consuming feed for no production. However, once-a-day milking is now being practised more widely in New Zealand for profit and lifestyle reasons. This is effective because the fall in milk yield is at least partially offset by labour and cost savings from milking once per day. This compares to some intensive farm systems in the United States that milk three or more times per day due to higher milk yields per cow and lower marginal labour costs.

Farmers who are contracted to supply liquid milk for human consumption often have to manage their herd so that the contracted number of cows is in milk the year round or the required minimum milk output is maintained. This is done by mating cows outside their natural mating time so that the period when each cow in the herd is giving maximum production is in rotation throughout the year.

Northern hemisphere farmers who keep cows in barns almost all the year usually manage their herds to give continuous production of milk so that they get paid all year round. In the southern hemisphere the cooperative dairying systems allow for two months on no productivity because their systems are designed to take advantage of maximum grass and milk production in the spring and because the milk processing plants pay bonuses in the dry (winter) season to carry the farmers through the mid-winter break from milking.

It also means that cows have a rest from milk production when they are most heavily pregnant. Some year-round milk farms are penalised financially for over-production at any time in the year by being unable to sell their overproduction at current prices.

INDIA'S TRADITIONAL DAIRY PRODUCTS

From burfi to kulfi, from *kalakand* to *shrikhand,* from *gulabjamun* to *chumchum* extends the delectable world of Indian milk delicacies. This article brings together information culled from diverse sources on age-old, milk-based specialties from different regions. Also included is information culled from diverse sources on the Indian milk-based sweets and other specialties from different regions of the country.

Since time immemorial, a significant proportion of milk has been used in India for preparing a wide variety of dairy delicacies — an unending array of sweets and other specialties from different regions of the country. In the process, the basic limitation of milk — its perishable nature — has been tastefully overcome. Its processing aims to extend the shelf-life of milk, while converting it into mouth-watering tit-bits.

Thus, diverse methods to prepare as well as preserve milk products have been developed. An estimated 50 to 55 per cent of the milk produced in India is converted into a variety of traditional milk products, using processes such as coagulation (heat and/or acid), desiccation and fermentation. Over the millennia, these processes have largely remained unchanged, being in the hands of halwais, the traditional sweetmeat makers, who form the core of this cottage industry.

Although 46 per cent of the milk produced in the country is consumed as liquid milk, increase in consumption can be stimulated. Milk plays an important role in the national diet. In Indian households, the life of milk is extended from 12 to 24 hours by repeated boiling. It is preserved by souring with the aid of lactic cultures, which imparts an acid taste, particularly refreshing in hot climate.

Curd

The first of these products developed was *dahi* (curds or yogurt), obtained by fermenting milk. In the process, the digestibility of milk constituents improves.The product is widely consumed along with meals. The surplus dahi is used as the intermediate product and churned into *makkhan* (butter), while the liquid whey — *chhach* or *mattha*— is consumed as a refreshing beverage or converted into *kadhi,* a spicy dish served hot with rice.

Nutritional benefits: When food is supplemented with 250 gms of dahi a day, the status of thiamine improves. *Dahi* also increases the pyruvic and lactic acids among children on a typical poor rice diet. Due to fermentation of milk, a greater amount of phosphorus and calcium is made available to the digestive system by their precipitation in the lower intestines due to the acid condition induced by Lactobacillus sp. The consumption of sour milk also results in increased efficiency of the human body to cope with a sudden influx of lactic acid in the system.

Dahi can also be consumed by people who suffer from lactose intolerance. Thus, dahi in its different forms as lassi, kadhi, shrikhand, etc. also contributes significantly to improve the nutritive contents of an average Indian diet.

Ghee and Makkhan

A week's collection of makkhan(butter) is converted into *ghee. Dahi* has a shelf-life of a day or two; *makkhan,* a week; and *ghee,* about a year. Ghee, thus, became the main dairy product for extended preservation. A system of collection of ghee from villages for trade gradually developed. Ghee mandis (trading centers) have been in existence for centuries. India produces some 900,000 tonnes of *ghee,* valued at Rs 85,000 million.The value of the resultant *lassi* is Rs 25,000 million.

For most uses, the wholesome flavour of *ghee* is its chief attraction. It is served in melted form and mixed with rice or lightly spread on *chappatis*. It is widely used for shallow frying and deep frying of food. Innumerable Indian sweetmeats based on cereals, milk solids, fruits and vegetables are cooked, by preference, in ghee.

Butter-milk is a by-product in the preparation of *makkhan*. It is estimated that about 55 kg of butter-milk is produced for every kg of ghee. While most of it is consumed by villagers and their families, some quantity is either given away or fed to cattle. The reason for this is lack of any market for it in rural areas. Butter-milk is rich in milk protein and calcium, and forms a nutritive and refreshing beverage.

Nutritional benefits: Makkhan and ghee contribute as much as one-third of the fat in the Indian diet. Ghee is produced mainly for consumption directly as food and as an ingredient of food preparations including sweets. Over the centuries, people have cultivated a liking for the aroma and flavour of ghee and prefer it over vegetable oils, the other traditional cooking medium. The vegetarian habits of many Indians preclude from their diet animal fats such as tallow or lard, used in the West.

Thus, ghee forms an important source of fat in the vegetarian diet. *Ghee* and *makkhan* are important sources of vitamins A, D, E and K. They also contain small amounts of essential fatty acids such as arachidonic and linoleic. Considerable losses of Vitamin A and carotene can occur during cooking, the latter being more rapid. Below 125°C, Vitamin A is fairly stable, but above this temperature it is rapidly destroyed. Some 10-20 per cent of carotene is lost during the normal cooking operations.

Khoa and Chhana

One major milk product in common use is *khoa,* obtained by rapidly evaporating milk in shallow pans to a total solids of about 70 per cent and capable of being preserved as such for several days. It is used as an ingredient in making different kinds of traditional mithais (sweets) such as *peda, burfi* and *gulabjamun*. Some 900,000 tonnes of khoa valued at Rs 45,000 million is produced in the country.

Yet another milk product of significance is *chhana,* a product of acid coagulation of hot milk and draining out of whey. It is used in preparing different kinds of sweets such as rasagollas. As they are especially popular in the Eastern region, they are called Bengali sweets. Approximately 1,200,000 tonnes of chhana, valued at Rs 6,000 million is produced in India.

The value of khoa and chhana produced is probably twice the value of all milk handled by the organized sector in the country. The traditional dairy products sector in India, like its agricultural counterpart, is grossly undermanaged. It, however, provides economic opportunities that even the Western dairy world would be envious of. The value of khoa and chhana-based sweets could possibly exceed Rs 130,000 million. India's high-value, high-volume market for traditional dairy products and delicacies is all set to boom further under the technology of mass production. This market is the largest in value after liquid milk and is estimated at US $3 billion in India and US $1 billion overseas. More and more dairy plants in the public, cooperative and private sectors in India are going in for the manufacture of traditional milk products.

This trend will undoubtedly give a further stimulus to the milk consumption in the country and ensure a better price to primary milk producers. Simultaneously, it will also help to productively utilize India's growing milk surplus.

Eggs as Dairy

Eggs are sometimes categorized as dairy, defining dairy as "food that is produced by animals (other than meat)" rather than as milk specifically. The Open Directory Project at one point listed cooking eggs as a subcategory of cooking dairy products. Defining dairy as limited to milk products, however, is more common.

Industrial Product

Cream and Butter

Today, milk is separated by large machines in bulk into cream and skim milk. The cream is processed to produce various consumer products, depending on its thickness, its suitability for culinary uses and consumer demand, which differs from place to place and country to country. Some cream is dried and powdered, some is condensed (by evaporation) mixed with varying amounts of sugar and canned. Most cream from New Zealand and Australian factories is made into butter.

This is done by churning the cream until the fat globules coagulate and form a monolithic mass. This butter mass is washed and, sometimes, salted to improve keeping qualities. The residual buttermilk goes on to further processing. The butter is packaged (25 to 50 kg boxes) and chilled for storage and sale. At a later stage these packages are broken down into home-consumption sized packs. Butter sells for about US$3200 a tonne on the international market in 2007 (an unusual high).

Skim Milk

The product left after the cream is removed is called skim, or skimmed, milk. Reacting skim milk with rennet or with an acid makes casein curds from the milk solids in skim milk, with whey as a residual. To make a consumable liquid a portion of cream is returned to the skim milk to make *low fat milk* (semi-skimmed) for human consumption. By varying the amount of cream returned, producers can make a variety of low-fat milks to suit their local market. Other products, such as calcium, vitamin D, and flavouring, are also added to appeal to consumers.

Casein

Casein is the predominant phosphoprotein found in fresh milk. It has a very wide range of uses from being a filler for human foods, such as in ice cream, to the manufacture of products such as fabric, adhesives, and plastics.

Cheese

Cheese is another product made from milk. Whole milk is reacted to form curds that can be compressed, processed and stored to form cheese. In countries where milk is legally allowed to be processed without pasteurisation a wide range of cheeses can be made using the bacteria naturally in the milk. In most other countries, the range of cheeses is smaller and the use of artificial cheese curing is greater. Whey is also the byproduct of this process.

Cheese has historically been an important way of "storing" milk over the year, and carrying over its nutritional value between prosperous years and fallow ones. It is a food product that, with bread and beer, dates back to prehistory in Middle Eastern and European cultures, and like them is subject to innumerable variety and local specificity. Although nowhere near as big as the market for cow's milk cheese, a considerable amount of cheese is made commercially from other milks, especially goat and sheep.

Whey

In earlier times whey was considered to be a waste product and it was, mostly, fed to pigs as a convenient means of disposal. Beginning about 1950, and mostly since about 1980, lactose and many other products, mainly food additives, are made from both casein and cheese whey.

Yogurt

Yoghurt making is a process similar to cheese making; only the process is arrested before the curd becomes very hard.

Milk Powders

Milk is also processed by various drying processes into powders. Whole milk and skim-milk powders for human and animal consumption and buttermilk (the residue from butter-making) powder is used for animal food.

The main difference between production of powders for human or for animal consumption is in the protection of the process and the product from contamination. Some people drink milk reconstituted from powdered milk, because milk is about 88 per cent water and it is much cheaper to transport the dried product. Dried skim milk powder is worth about US$5300 a tonne (mid-2007 prices) on the international market.

Other Milk Products

Kumis is produced commercially in Central Asia. Although it is traditionally made from mare's milk, modern industrial variants may use cow's milk instead.

TRANSPORT OF MILK

Historically, the milking and the processing took place in the same place: on a dairy farm. Later, cream was separated from the milk by machine, on the farm, and the cream was transported to a factory for butter making. The skim milk was fed to pigs. This allowed for the high cost of transport (taking the smallest volume high-value product), primitive trucks and the poor quality of roads.

Only farms close to factories could afford to take whole milk, which was essential for cheese making in industrial quantities, to them. The development of refrigeration and better road transport, in the late 1950s, has meant that most farmers milk their cows and only temporarily store the milk in large refrigerated bulk tanks, whence it is later transported by truck to central processing facilities.

MILKING MACHINE

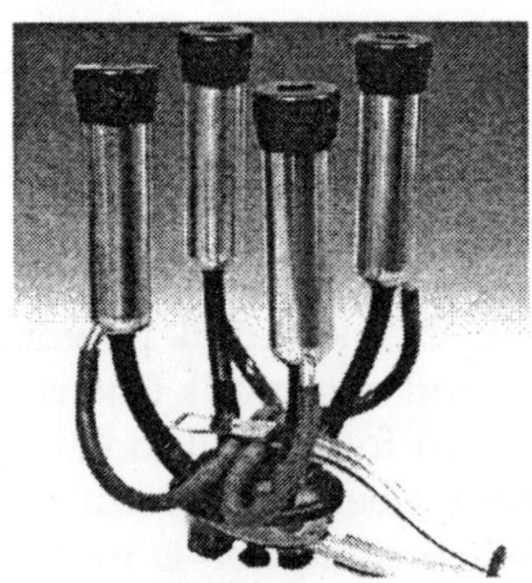

Fig. Milking Machine.

The milking machine is a nearly automatic machine installation for milking cows. It is not a single unit, but rather an assembly of components designed to handle as many as 200 cows an hour. The system consists of the cluster (the assembly that is manually attached to the cow), a milk tube, a pulse tube and pulsator, a vacuum pump or blower, and perhaps a recorder jar or milk meter that measures yield. Together, the system allows milk to flow into a pipeline in preparation for shipping to a processing plant.

The cluster consists of teatcups, a shell and liner device that actually performs the milking action, and a claw or manifold that spaces the teatcups and connects them to the milk and pulse tubes. The milk tube carries the milk and air mixture away from the cow's udder to receiving tanks. The pulse tube, or airline, carries the varying air pressure from the pulsator device to the tanks, drawing the milk and fluids out of the cows as well. In operation, milk is drawn from the cow's teats because a vacuum is created within the cup device, forcing the milk through the teat canal. The pulsator alternates the pressure, first creating a vacuum (milk phase), and then applying air, which causes the flexible liner in the cup to collapse and massage the teat (rest phase). The alternating process of milk-and-rest is continued in a rhythmic pattern for the cows' health and good milk productivity.

Early attempts at milking cows involved a variety of methods. Around 380 B.C., Egyptians, along with traditional milking-by-hand, inserted wheat straws into cows' teats. Suction was first used as a basis for the mechanized harvesting of milk in 1851, although the attempts were not altogether successful, drawing too much blood and body fluid congestion within the teat.

To encourage further innovations, the Royal Agricultural Society of England offered money for a safe, working milking machine. Around the 1890s Alexander Shiels of Glasgow, Scotland, developed a pulsator that alternated suction levels to successfully massage the blood and fluids out of the teat for proper blood circulation. That device, along with the development of a double-chambered teatcup in 1892, led to milking machines replacing hand milking. After the 1920s machine milking became firmly established in the dairy industry. Today, the majority of all milking is processed by machine.

THE MANUFACTURING PROCESS

The milking machine components are created and assembled in several major manufacturing plants throughout the world using traditional processes and procedures. Stainless steel and plastic are used for containers and liners and cast iron and steel for vacuum pumps, controls, and metering devices.

Receiving

Here stainless steel is received in large sheet or tube form. Stainless steel is used to fabricate components that will come in contact with milk. The sheets are protected from scratches by a vinyl lining, which will be removed later after forming and machining. Milking machine components are created using stainless steel and plastic for containers and liners, and cast iron and steel for vacuum pumps, controls, and metering devices. At this point, the stainless steel from the foundry has a dull finish.

Cutting, Machining and Forming

The steel sheets may be sent directly to a polishing station where large machines create a smooth finish. Once the initial finish is achieved, the sheets may move on rollers to numerically controlled punch machines, where they are cut into shapes for various parts. From there, some parts are formed or bent into shape on large brakes. Mounting panels for controls, structural components, and small detail parts for the claws and pumps are made at this stage.

Creating the Shell and Claws

The shell that contains the liner is fabricated as an extrusion. This process involves forcing steel tubing over a die under heat and pressure to form the elongated rigid piece. The claw is made as a series of smaller extruded pieces of tubing that form the manifold, which spaces the teatcups in a cluster formation. The extrusions are then manually welded together in fixtures according to the desired size. Both the completed claws and shell have a dull finish that will require polishing.

Making the Receivers

Receiver tanks are stainless steel tanks that receive milk from the milk lines, generally holding from 15-26 gallons (60-100 1). Although some are customised plastic, most are steel with the heads or ends spun on specialty machines. This production technique shapes a thin steel disc as it is being turned in a lathe. The disc is shaped as it is forced over a steel shape or mandrel.

Once the operator forms the ends of the receiver as cups, another technician will weld the body to the head, leaving orifices or openings for milk input and output. Individually manufactured, the receivers will also be polished by hand. Some receivers will have translucent plastic panel inserts so that dairy farmers can visually gauge the cow's milk production.

Polishing

All major stainless steel components are polished to the familiar finish associated with food-handling equipment. The manufacturers use a variety of mechanized belts, cloths, and spinning wheels in what becomes a very labour intensive process to meet government and industry sanitary standards.

This polishing is in addition to the polishing the large stainless sheets undergo following receiving. Workers wield an assortment of hand polishers and attachments to shine all contact and protective surfaces, from the claws to receivers to pipelines.

Making the Vacuum Pumps or Blowers

These "drivers" of air and fluids through the system are manufactured by select vendors. The unit is basically a sealed iron case with a set of timing gears inside and an impeller, resembling two blades or paddles on a shaft, that spins at over 3,000 revolutions per minute to create a vacuum that will draw fluids in the line. The making of the pumps requires raw castings to be poured for the various parts. The rough parts are hand-machined on a bench by technicians and then placed on a CNC rotating cutter table where the cutting stone makes two precise passes along the pre-determined edges to cut away any rough surfaces.

The assembly of the major components—along with seals, bearings, and shafts—is critical because a variation of just 0.002 inch can change the balance and affect the pump. The components are placed on a coordinate measuring machine where the profile is checked so that all parts fit properly. The technicians, using feeler gauges, will set proper clearances before locking the critical gear parts in place and bolting the unit together. Then they will run the pumps in a test booth before releasing them for distribution.

Assembly

The manufactured and purchased parts are placed in several different areas where the milking machine subassemblies come together. Technicians will select the parts according to the system design specifications, often customised to meet certain operations. It is at this stage that pressures and loads will gauge equipment performance. Final assembly of all machine components will not occur until after shipment to the farm and installation in bams, where often elaborate stalls and stations will be used to maximize the milk harvest.

Workers at assembly will also make initial line connections from valves to pumps to meters, checking for tolerances and poor fits. Vacuum pumps or blowers, the heart of the milking system, are tested so that both milk and accompanying air can be efficiently removed. The pumps will be tested under simulated loads.

Vacuum controllers, which admit the necessary air to maintain the proper vacuum level, are selected. The air lines and milk lines are selected to size and connection hardware grouped. Controls, also purchased, are prepared for installation.

STANDARDS

Milking machine manufacturers are subject to a variety of standards, some self-imposed. In addition to inspections throughout the manufacturing process, all installations are set up by trained dealers and electrical contractors. Equipment designers follow Association of Agricultural Engineer standards and sanitary guidelines established by a dairy industry council.

The Future

Advances in technology have introduced several new innovations to milking machines. Automatic detacher units that connect loosely to the milking claw allow cows to move and shift freely during milking. Based on the rate of milk flow, the detacher can also detect the end of milking, shutting the vacuum and actually removing the claw from the cow.

Automatic backflushing units are also gaining popularity. These units and systems send chemical and rinse solutions through pipelines and clusters to reduce the risk of infection and mastitis (udder inflammation).

The use of automatic identification systems, such as electronic transponder cow neck-tags, have enabled dairy farmers to keep track of milk production by individual cows.

Robotics are at the forefront of milking technology, especially in Europe. Automatic attachment devices have been created but not quite perfected. This new innovation will require little manual labour, and the machines will oversee much of the milking process from the time a cow enters a milking centre until it leaves to graze.

Milking Shed Layouts

Bail-style sheds: This type of milking facility was the first development, after open-paddock milking, for many farmers. The building was a long, narrow, *lean-to* shed that was open along one long side. The cows were held in a yard at the open side and when they were about to be milked they were positioned in one of the bails (stalls). Usually the cows were restrained in the bail with a breech chain and a rope to restrain the outer back leg.

The cow could not move about excessively and the milker could expect not to be kicked or trampled while sitting on a stool and milking into a bucket. When each cow was finished she backed out into the yard again. As herd sizes increased a door was set into the front of each bail so that when the milking was done for any cow the milker could, after undoing the leg-rope and with a remote link, open the door and allow her to exit to the pasture. The door was closed; the next cow walked into the bail and was secured. When milking machines were introduced bails were set in pairs so that a cow was being milked in one paired bail while the other could be prepared for milking.

When one was finished the machine's cups are swapped to the other cow. This is the same as for *Swingover Milking Parlours* as described below except that the cups are loaded on the udder from the side. As herd numbers increased it was easier to double-up the cup-sets and milk both cows simultaneously than to increase the number of bails. About 50 cows an hour can be milked in a shed with 8 bales by one person.

Herringbone Milking Parlours: In herringbone milking sheds, or parlours, cows enter, in single file, and line up almost perpendicular to the central aisle of the milking parlour on both sides of a central pit in which the milker works. After washing the udder and teats the cups of the milking machine are applied to the cows, from the rear of their hind legs, on both sides of the working area. Large herringbone sheds can milk up to 600 cows efficiently with two people.

Swingover Milking Parlours: Swingover parlours are the same as herringbone parlours except they have only one set of milking cups to be shared between the two rows of cows, as one side is being milked the cows on the other side are moved out and replaced with unmilked ones. The advantage of this system is that it is less costly to equip, however it operates at slightly better than half-speed and one would not normally try to milk more than about 100 cows with one person.

Rotary Milking Sheds: Rotary milking sheds consist of a turntable with about 12 to 100 individual stalls for cows around the outer edge. A "good" rotary will be operated with 24–32 stalls by one (two) milkers. The turntable is turned by an electric-motor drive at a rate that one turn is the time for a cow to be milked completely. As an empty stall passes the entrance a cow steps on, facing the centre, and rotates with the turntable. The next cow moves into the next vacant stall and so on.

The operator, or milker, cleans the teats, attaches the cups and does any other feeding or whatever husbanding operations that is necessary. Cows are milked as the platform rotates. The milker, or an automatic device, removes the milking machine cups and the cow backs out and leaves at an exit just before the entrance. The rotary system is capable of milking very large herds—over a thousand cows.

Automatic Milking sheds: Automatic milking or 'robotic milking' sheds can be seen in many European countries. Current automatic milking sheds use the voluntary milking (VM) method. These allow the cows to voluntarily present themselves for milking at any time of the day or night, although repeat visits may be limited by the farmer through computer software. A robot arm is used to clean teats and apply milking equipment, while automated gates direct cow traffic, eliminating the need for the farmer to be present during the process. The entire process is computer controlled. There is a description of an automatic system here—

Supplementary accessories in sheds: Farmers soon realised that a milking shed was a good place to feed cows supplementary foods that overcame local dietary deficiencies or added to the cows' wellbeing and production. Each bail might have a box into which such feed is delivered as the cow arrives so that she is eating while being milked. A computer can read the eartag of each beast to ration the correct individual supplement.

The holding yard at the entrance of the shed is important as a means of keeping cows moving into the shed. Most yards have a powered gate that ensures that the cows are kept close to the shed. Water is a vital commodity on a dairy farm: cows drink about 20 gallons (80 litres) a day, sheds need water to cool and clean them. Pumps and reservoirs are common at milking facilities.

Chapter 8

Animal's Waste Management

Traditional small dairy farms effectively manage manure by applying it to their fields as a crop fertilizer. Unfortunately, Indian farm policy and economics are causing the demise of those small, diversified farms and the rise of industrial factory dairies that cram together thousands of cows who make millions of gallons of manure. One 2,500-cow dairy produces as much waste as a city with 400,000 residents.

Factory dairy operators often attempt to deal with the high volume of manure, as well as waste from the milking operation, by using water to flush it out of buildings and into multimillion-gallon lagoons. Then, the mixture is sprayed or spread onto fields to fertilize them. But unlike the relatively small amount of cow manure coming from traditional farms, these loads of industrial dairy waste are too much for the land to absorb and filter. Instead, the manure pollutes the air, water, and soil. It also causes human health problems.

Storing millions of gallons of manure and other waste in one place emits dust particles and hundreds of different volatile gases, including ammonia, carbon dioxide and methane. In fact, two California industrial dairy workers died in 2001 from methane overexposure while they were working in a 30-foot deep manure pit. The dairy foreman and the manager were indicted for involuntary manslaughter over the deaths in February 2003. In addition to methane, the lagoons give off hydrogen sulfide, which can cause brain damage. It threatens the safety of workers and people living nearby.

Manure from factory dairies also poisons waterways and wells when, a lagoon wall collapses, an operator fails to handle pumps properly, or the waste spills out of lagoons during heavy rains.

Manure contains nitrates and phosphorus. When too many of these nutrients enter waterways, they prompt the rapid growth of algae and other aquatic plants that consume much of the oxygen in the water. This smothers fish and other animals and causes serious taste and odor problems in drinking water.

Each state issues permits that allow factory dairies and other confined animal feeding operations to operate. Regulators issue relatively few fines and rarely shut down the dairies because of spills or other pollution problems.

In countries where cows are grazed outside year-round there is little waste disposal to deal with. The most concentrated waste is at the milking shed where the animal waste is liquefied (during the water-washing process) and allowed to flow by gravity, or pumped, into composting ponds with anaerobic bacteria to consume the solids. The processed water and nutrients are then pumped back onto the pasture as irrigation and fertilizer. Surplus animals are slaughtered for processed meat and other rendered products.

In the associated milk processing factories most of the waste is washing water that is treated, usually by composting, and returned to waterways. This is much different from half a century ago when the main products were butter, cheese and casein, and the rest of the milk had to be disposed of as waste (sometimes as animal feed).

In areas where cows are housed all year round the waste problem is difficult because of the amount of feed that is bought in and the amount of bedding material that also has to be removed and composted. The size of the problem can be understood by standing downwind of the barns where such dairying goes on.

In many cases modern farms have very large quantities of milk to be transported to a factory for processing. If anything goes wrong with the milking, transport or processing facilities it can be a major disaster trying to dispose of enormous quantities of milk. If a road tanker overturns on a road the rescue crew is looking at accommodating the spill of 10 to 20 thousand gallons of milk without allowing any into the waterways. A derailed rail tanker-train may involve 10 times that amount. Without refrigeration, milk is a fragile commodity and it is very damaging to the environment in its raw state. A widespread electrical power blackout is another disaster for the dairy industry because both milking and processing facilities are affected.

In dairy-intensive areas the simplest way of disposing of large quantities of milk has been to dig a large hole in the ground and allow the clay to filter the milk solids as it soaks away. This is not very satisfactory.

DAIRY MANURE MANAGEMENT

Dairy manure management can be classified into three systems — solid, slurry or lagoon — depending on the collection, transportation and distribution of manure on the fields. These systems are dependent on the amount of bedding and water dilution used by a specific operation. Many dairies use more than one system. Manure from dry cows and replacement heifers may be handled as a solid, whereas manure from free-stall barns, holding pens and milking parlors may be handled as a liquid, or solids may be separated from the liquid wastes so it can be used for other purposes.

Solid systems are commonly used in smaller operations (less than 100 cows) with bedded loafing barns or stanchion stalls. These systems minimize the volume of manure that is handled; however, a separate facility is required for liquid milking centre manure.

Slurry systems maximize recovery of plant nutrients from manure and are often used where geologic conditions are unsuitable for a lagoon system. These systems increase the volume of manure to be handled because of the higher water content, but allow the manure to be handled as a fluid. Many dairies favour lagoon systems because costs are lower than for other systems. Lagoons are applicable where flushing is desired and where a significant amount of lot runoff must be contained.

To minimize pollution potential and maximize nutrient recovery, incorporate livestock manure into the soil as soon as possible after application. To prevent applying an excess of plant nutrients (N, P and K), keep long-term records on the amount applied to each field. Make an analysis to determine the nutrient content of the manure and keep an estimate of the amount of manure applied. The amount of land required for manure disposal is usually based on 100 pounds of nitrogen used annually for plant production per acre.

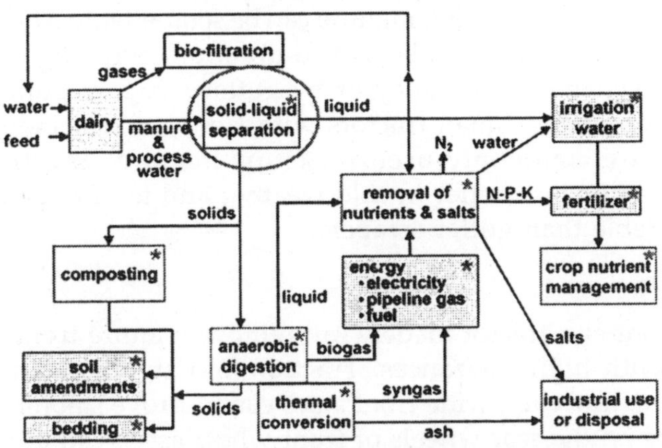

Fig. Dairy Waste Management

Consult local health and regulatory authorities and have all plans approved before constructing any manure handling system. A dairy operation with 700 or more cows is required by state law to obtain a permit. Any livestock manure management system, regardless of size, must be designed and operated in a manner that will not pollute surface or groundwater.

Local Extension centre or Natural Resources Conservation Service (NRCS) office may be contacted for information about permits and assistance in developing manure management systems.

SOLID WASTE SYSTEMS

Manure with a 75 to 80 percent moisture content can

usually be handled as a solid. Manure at this moisture content has a consistency of peanut butter. Dairy manure, as excreted, contains about 88 percent water. So, to be handled as a solid, dairy manure must have the liquids drained off or bedding added. Twelve pounds of bedding per 100 pounds of fresh manure (about 4 pounds of dry straw per cow per day) is needed to permit handling dairy manure as a solid.

Scraping Systems

Manure from bedded housing usually has to be handled as a solid. As a semisolid, manure can be scraped into a holding area where liquids are allowed to drain off. Scraping can be done mechanically by alley or by gutter scrapers pulled by cables or chains. Small tractors with front- or rear-mounted blades are commonly used to scrape manure, and tractor scrapers function better in cold weather and tend to be more dependable than gutter scrapers.

Loaders

Front-end tractor loaders can remove manure from large areas with high clearances. Traction and stability can be a problem, however; wide front axles can improve stability and weights on the rear wheels or front-wheel-assist can improve traction. Skid steer loaders can work in cramped quarters and, in general, lessen time and hand labour expended.

Manure Storage

Storage is required with most solid handling systems because of weather or limited available fields. A 60-day minimum storage capacity is recommended. The storage area should have all-weather access with surface runoff water diverted from the storage area. Any draining liquid should be directed to a soil-plant filter, lagoon or holding pond. A roof can eliminate the need for collecting and storing runoff from the storage area.

Manure Spreaders

Most solid manure manure spreaders have moving aprons

to move the load rearward to beaters. Flail-type spreaders have chains attached to a shaft that revolves at high speed to flail the manure out of the tank. These spreaders are also suited for semisolid manure.

SLURRY WASTE SYSTEMS

Manure with 90 to 96 percent moisture content can usually be handled as a fluid but may require special pumps. Manure at this moisture content has the consistency of malt. Manure with 96 to 98 percent water content can be handled with ordinary pumps and flushing equipment if excessive straw or fibrous material is not present. For conventional pumping, two gallons of water must be added to dilute a gallon of fresh manure to 96 percent. Of course, this greatly increases the volume of manure to be stored and transported.

Flushing is not well suited to a slurry manure management system. The slurry system is designed to minimize dilution because it uses tank wagons for transportation and application. Therefore, hauling extra water with the manure is not profitable.

Assume a 1400-pound cow produces 14 gallons of undiluted manure per day. Hauling her yearly manure output will require 1.7 trips to the field with a 3,000-gallon tank wagon. If manure is diluted to 4 percent solids, 5.1 trips per cow per year will be required.

Slurry Manure Storage

Slurry can be stored in earthen basins, below-ground and above-ground concrete tanks and in lined and unlined metal tanks. Slurry storage areas are usually designed for a 120-day minimum storage capacity. In some locations, soil type can prohibit the use of earthen basins or require the use of a membrane-type liner. In these locations, concrete or steel manure storage tanks may be used.

Depending on the location of buildings and lots, it may be possible to gravity drain or scrape manure into the storage structure. In-ground tanks must be designed to resist lateral forces from the soil when the tank is empty. Outside drainage may be necessary to prevent the tank from floating when it is empty and the soil is saturated. Most above-ground tanks have the added expense of a pump to transfer manure in and out of the facility.

Earth Basins

Earth basins are usually partially below the original grade and partially above. The above-ground berms divert surface runoff water from the basin. Check with the Division of Geology and Land Survey for suitable sites, soil suitability and construction details to avoid seepage polluting surface water or groundwater. Earthen basins must be constructed with a clay seal (bottom and sides) to prevent leakage. In some cases, an artificial liner may be required. If soils have a high potential for collapsing, MDNR will not approve an earthen manure storage structure. In these cases, an alternate site must be selected, or a concrete or steel tank used for storage.

Scrape to Storage

Scraping into below-ground storage areas can reduce equipment investment and maintenance costs. Any system that involves uncovered concrete lots, alleys or exercise areas increases the amount of runoff water that is hauled. Above-ground tanks require scraping into a collection pit and then pumping.

Pumps

Pumps are frequently used to move manure into tanks and to move manure from tanks into tank wagons. High capacity (1,000 to 3,000 gpm) chopper pumps are used to move dairy manure from storage, with extra capacity to mix solids and liquids.

Tank Wagons

Tractor-drawn tank wagons have capacities from 1,000 to 3,000 gallons. For long hauls and/or large operations, a tank truck may be more economical. Tank wagons can either spread the liquid on the soil or be equipped with knives to inject the manure into the soil. Injection reduces odors and nitrogen loss but requires considerable power to pull the tank wagon and injectors at a reasonable speed.

Injection can not be done when the soil is frozen or if it is too rocky. Likewise, spreading manure on frozen soil could pollute surface water if it rains or snows while the ground is still frozen.

Slurry manure systems require more land for application than lagoon systems because more nitrogen is retained.

LAGOON WASTE SYSTEMS

Lagoon systems handle highly diluted manure (96 percent or more water) that can be pumped through irrigation systems. Most lagoon effluent is more than 99 percent water, so it has the consistency of water.

Flushing is the preferred method of manure collection and transportation for many dairies because it eliminates the labour required for scraping and moving manure to storage. Lagoons complement flushing systems because they provide storage at relatively low cost and usually do not cause unacceptable odor problems if judiciously located. Lagoons can also provide a source of flush water.

The anaerobic breakdown of manure usually results in acceptable odor levels when applied by an irrigation system. Approximately 90 percent of the input nitrogen is lost or unavailable in an unagitated lagoon, but this can be an advantage if limited land is available for manure disposal. For large operations, lagoons provide the least-cost alternative on a per-cow basis.

Consideration should be given to separating fibrous material (free-stall bedding, wasted hay, silage, etc.) from the manure flow going to the lagoon. Experience has shown that excessive amounts of this material can build up as surface crust and increase the rate of sludge accumulation in the lagoon, thus decreasing its long-term effectiveness as a manure storage and treatment facility.

Lagoons are usually designed for a 365-day storage capacity with all manure going into the lagoon. This includes dry cow manure, but not calf and replacement heifer manure. Also note that lagoons are not allowed by MDNR in areas where soil collapse potential is high.

Lagoons are usually formed by excavation and above-ground berms. The berms divert surface runoff water from the lagoon, but a diversion channel may be required. For a "DNR approved system," a clay seal (compacted by a sheepsfoot roller) must be on the bottom and sides to meet NRCS specifications. Also, lagoons must be filled with fresh water to the minimum operating level and the berms seeded and mulched prior to operation.

Pumps

Conventional irrigation pumps are adequate for pumping lagoons if the intake is floated about 1 to 2 feet below the surface. The floating intake prevents surface debris interference and reduces the handling of sludge.

Centrifugal power-take-off irrigation pumps are a practical alternative for irrigating from lagoons. Small engine-mounted low-lift pumps can also provide adequate capacity and pressure to pump a small lagoon.

A complete manure management system includes a way of spreading manure in a pollution-free manner. It is important that all irrigation systems be monitored while effluent is being applied so no runoff occurs at the application site. The following are ways to spread manure:

Surface Irrigation Systems

Gated pipe can provide a low-cost distribution system for pumping small lagoons, especially where uniform application is not critical. Small systems can use a "homemade" gated pipe made from polyethylene pipe (e.g., using 2-inch diameter pipe for 50 gpm systems) with holes in the pipe at 30- to 40-inch intervals.

The holes must be small enough that flow is distributed out of all of the holes, but large enough that they don't become clogged by small solids. These systems are feasible for small lagoons handling only milkhouse manure but have been used for larger lagoons. For larger systems, commercial gated pipe with adjustable gates is an alternative.

Sprinkler Irrigation Systems

For irregular rolling land, use a sprinkler irrigation system instead of gated pipe. Various sprinkler systems are suitable; the choice depends on the desire to save labour or money.

Stationary Hand-carried Systems

For small operations, one or more small sprinklers fed by 3- to 6-inch portable pipe is adequate if time and labour are available. For even smaller operations, a 1 DA 2- to 1-inch nozzle sprinkler(s), covering 1 DA 2 to 2 acres per set, can be used. For larger operations, a high volume gun sprinkler with a 1- to 2-inch nozzle, covering 2 1 DA 2 to 6 acres per set, can be used to reduce labour requirement.

Moving Sprinkler Systems

To reduce labour and to accommodate larger operations, a traveling gun or a centre-pivot irrigator may be more cost-effective than hand-moved sprinklers. Different models of the small traveling guns are now available. Larger traveling guns, used for crop irrigation, can be used if crops are irrigated conventionally or if rental units are available.

DAIRY MANURE MANAGEMENT

Concerns regarding nutrient losses from the manure of large dairy herds to groundwater or surface runoff have been extremely acute in Florida. The most widely publicized concerns have been with phosphorus (P) contamination of Lake Okeechobee, probably washing off the farms in surface runoff during the summer rainy season. Also of concern are nitrogen (N) losses in the form of nitrate into the groundwater through the deep sandy soils of the Suwannee River basin.

Florida is not unique. All states are starting to monitor farms where large numbers of food-producing animals are maintained on small acreage. But regardless of farm size, maintenance of the environment and efficient utilization of nutrients should be a priority. Nitrogen (N) and phosphorus (P) are the primary nutrients of concern. Manure N can be converted to nitrates in the soil and potentially leach to groundwater.

Manure P can potentially move with surface runoff, thus stimulating algae and aquatic plant growth leading to eutrophication of surface waters. Potassium (K) has not been of as much concern environmentally as N and P, but it is of equal concern in fertilizer management strategies. Also, K is important in assessing equivalent commercial fertilizer value of manure. Manure nutrients and decaying organic matter are natural components of the environment that ultimately contribute to the production of more plant and animal tissue. Thus, concern about manure leakage is no different than concern about commercial fertilizer use. Manure is in fact a resource, based largely on its equivalence with commercial fertilizer, and should not be called a waste when it is recycled through new plant growth.

To use the resource value of manure effectively and to avoid excessive concentration of these nutrients at inappropriate points, it is helpful to budget nutrient flow through the total dairy farm system. If there is a problem concentration at some point, then corrective measures can be taken which are environmentally accountable.

This publication is designed to give background information and serve as a guide to dairy farmers and planners to help develop answers to these questions for an individual dairy farm.

Abbreviations: N = nitrogen, P = phosphorus, K = potassium, CP = crude protein, DM = dry matter, DMI = DM intake, Mcal = megacalorie of energy, NE_L = net energy for lactation, OM = organic matter, TDN = total digestible nutrients.

Individual Nutrientsis Excreted by Dairy Cow

Historically, the nutrient excretion standards most often used in the design of manure management systems were those of the American Society of Agricultural Engineers. These standards are based on body weight of cows, however, they do not account for the large variation among dairies in nutrient excretion levels. The variation is caused by differing voluntary feed intake, differing supplemental levels, and differing amounts of nutrients harvested in the milk.

Recent University of Florida experiments showed that N and P excretions by dairy cows varied dramatically with level of N and P intakes. These data confirmed that excretion estimates for individual farms are best based on dietary intake of a nutrient minus the amount secreted into milk. Most dairy farms have accurate estimates of feed and milk and, thus, this method of predicting total excretion of minerals by dairy cows is used in this publication. The following milk composition, typical of Holsteins, was used along with pounds of milk to determine recovery of fed nutrients in milk:

- Protein3.30 per cent (N content.512 per cent)
- Phosphorus (P)0.10 per cent
- Calcium (Ca)0.12 per cent
- Potassium (K)0.15 per cent
- Magnesium (Mg)0.01 per cent
- Sodium (Na)0.05 per cent
- Chlorine (Cl)0.11 per cent

Dairy farmers have considerable control of mineral excretion because they control the mineral contents in the diets they feed. Feeding adequate P is important for animal health and performance. However,.40 per cent of total diet dry matter is near the year-round estimated requirements for lactating cows, more is recommended in early lactation.

Although these data do not lead us to recommend lowering feeding levels for P below standard feeding recommendations (NRC), the data point out that future committees that develop NRC feeding standards need to review recommended feeding levels for P, N, and environmentally sensitive minerals. The objective is to minimize excretion of these nutrients and still maintain optimum animal performance.

One is for cows consuming diets formulated to supply NRC crude protein standards which require more crude protein to assure that true protein needs are met (NRC, high). The other (NRC, low) minimizes dietary N by providing minimal nonprotein N and ruminally degradable protein for optimum rumen microbial fermentation and provides for remaining animal requirements with ruminally undegraded protein. Numeric estimates of yearly N excreted by high-producing 1400 lb cows were 273 lbs N per cow per year when fed according to the NRC crude protein standards and 234 lbs N per cow per year when diet protein was formulated for minimum needs for undegraded and degraded protein.

Diets designed to support higher milk production than many dairy farmers are currently achieving, most dairies with lower milk production choose to feed as much protein as was used in this example (e.g., up to 17.5 per cent crude protein of total diet dry matter for their high-producing group). Nutrient management plans usually should be based on current cow excretion estimates but, if expansion is planned, it may be helpful to estimate future needs as well.

To start, use current average production. If the herd averages 50 lbs of milk per day for all milking cows year-round (with dry cows managed on a separate farm), or if the herd averages 50 lbs year-round for all cows milking and dry (with dry cows managed in the same manure management system), then use excretion estimates for cows producing 50 lbs milk. Then multiply the excretion estimates by the average excretion per day for cows currently producing 50 lbs of milk per day by 365.

Significant volatilization of the N will occur because it is easily converted to ammonia and lost to the air as gaseous ammonia. Thus, fertilizer values will be somewhat less than amounts originally excreted. Although the value of N, P, and K fertilizer nutrients in manure usually will not be as great as the total costs of the waste management system, recovered value reduces the net cost of waste handling. However, value will be realised only if the nutrients in dairy manure are used to displace the purchase of inorganic fertilizer nutrients.

P—1.9 lbs actual P/ton wet manure (equivalent to 4.4 lbs P_2O_5)

K— 6.0 lbs actual K/ton wet manure (equivalent to 7.2 lbs K_2O)

Total solids 11.6 per cent

Manure composition changes as time passes after excretion. In addition to expected volatilization of N, liquids will drain from the solids, drying may occur, or the manure may be diluted with flushwater. Thus, the moisture content usually is quite different. It is important to take samples of manure or wastewater applied to cropland and have these samples analysed at a commercial laboratory. The analysis should include total Kjeldahl N and not just nitrate N, since almost no nitrate form of N occurs in manures. Nitrification does not occur until after manure is incorporated into the soil.

The major forms of N in dairy manure are either organic N or urea N which is easily converted to ammonia and can be lost to the air as gaseous ammonia.

Manure Management System

After excretion by the cow, manure may be stored wet, stored after being allowed to dry, flushed with water to a lagoon or holding pond, spread fresh on land, or spread in some form at some later time. The longer the time in storage, the greater the potential for N losses to the air as ammonia.

The greater the dilution with water, the greater the potential for nutrient losses to surface and groundwaters unless included as part of an irrigation programme to distribute water and nutrients to growing crops. Few manure systems on farms actually collect all of the feces and urine at one location for application to one particular unit of land.

Separations or losses occur in many ways.

- Flushed manure from the milking parlor and feed barn may go through a sand trap and be pumped over a separator screen before irrigation of land with the effluent.
- Manure is dropped in different areas such as pasture, milking parlor, cooling barns, and the primary feeding area and some of these "separations" may not be collectible for land-spreading.

- Some gaseous loss of ammonia occurs (volatilization) which returns a variable, but often controllable, portion of the N to the air.

Other possibilities include some surface runoff and loss to the groundwater. Management practices must control all of these components so that surface runoff and losses of nutrients to the groundwater are minimized and do not cause violations of state water quality standards.

The choice of a manure management system will depend on existing facilities. If the existing buildings were designed for flushing, then a dry handling system would not be possible without major structural modifications. If a new dairy is being planned, then other factors can be considered. In both cases, changes in the system must be compatible with other management practices on the dairy. The manure nutrients must be spread in a way that recovers nutrients in harvested crops or be stockpiled in a way that will not pose environmental risks before being spread.

Regulatory requirements may influence the choice of a waste management system. If surface runoff must be collected, stored, and dispersed on cropland, then a liquid handling system would be necessary. However, other components could still be handled as a solid or as slurry.

Types of Manure Handling Systems

Manure management systems can be categorized in many ways, with options within each type of system. The types of systems can be outlined as follows:

- Solid or conventional manure handling
- Slurry manure handling
- Liquid manure handling
- Anaerobic lagoon
- Removal of suspended solids
- Composting
- Combinations of the above

Each system can be broken down into five major components:

- Collection

- Storage
- Processing or treatment
- Transport
- Utilization

SOLID MANURE

Conventional or solid manure handling systems are not common in Florida. Normally high rainfall and humidity make it difficult to keep manure dry enough to be handled with a front-end loader. Also, the warmer climate permits the use of water for flushing on a year-round basis, as well as the utilization of wastewater on cropland in multiple cropping systems. Use of water for flushing of manure also has low labour requirements and is a clean way to handle manure.

Solid manure handling must employ some type of dry scraping for collection, and every effort must be made to keep out excess water. The manure can be hauled and spread on cropland on a daily basis or the manure can be placed in storage. The storage facility will require a roof or a provision must be made for capturing any liquid leachate or runoff in a pit or lagoon. Normally there would not be any processing or treatment of the manure. Transportation would probably be in a conventional box manure spreader, and utilization would be on cropland.

In Florida, a dairy farm would rarely attempt to employ a solid manure handling system for all of the manure. However, much of the manure can be handled as a solid. In the design of new or modified facilities, it is recommended that provisions be made for both scraping and/or flushing, if possible.

SLURRY MANURE

This is basically the mixture of excreted feces and urine with only enough water added to facilitate handling. This results in a solids content of greater than 5 per cent which is too wet to handle with a front-end loader but not dilute enough to handle in a conventional irrigation system. Storage could be in pits or in tanks either above or below ground. Transport would probably be in a tank truck or wagon or in a flail spreader. Utilization would be on cropland. If knifing or soil injection of manure nutrients is desired, this is the system of choice.

Use of slurry requires purchase of a tank truck or wagon, special pumps that will handle the high solids content, and construction of storage tanks that may be quite expensive. Loading, transporting, and spreading the slurry also has a high labour requirement but the system can result in low nutrient losses.

LIQUID MANURE HANDLING

This usually involves flush tanks to move manure and thus dilutes manure to a solids content of less than 5 per cent. In most Florida dairy systems, the solids content is less than 2 per cent and can be handled in specially designed irrigation equipment.

Required storage capacity depends on type of soils in the irrigation field, the storage time between irrigation applications, and the amount of stormwater runoff which the system must be capable of retaining. Some distinct advantages of this type of system are that it has low labour requirements and can result in relatively few nutrient losses when irrigation is frequent and growing crops are available to utilize the nutrients.

ANAEROBIC LAGOON SYSTEM

This system was the most popular type of manure handling system installed on Florida dairy farms during the 1970s and '80s. It actually is a specific type of liquid handling in which the flushed manure is directed into an anaerobic lagoon. The first stage of the lagoon system is designed with a constant liquid level to overflow into a second lagoon or pond designed for liquid storage capacity.

Effluent from the storage pond must be dispersed on cropland through some type of irrigation system. Although seepage irrigation and sheet flows have been used for effluent dispersal, pivot irrigation systems are becoming much more popular because of their even distribution of the manure nutrients. In addition to the effluent, sludge accumulates in the anaerobic lagoon which contains a significant amount of P and a small amount of the N. The amount of time before the lagoon fills with sludge to a point where it needs to be cleaned out varies depending on loading rates and design volume.

Cleanout of smaller, more heavily loaded lagoons every 2 to 5 years is common while larger lagoons may function much longer before cleanout is necessary. Separation of larger manure solids is often done prior to the wastewater entering the lagoon in order to permit accommodation of manure from more cows or to extend the time until cleanout is necessary.

Removal of Suspended Solids from Flushed Manure

Moving manure from animal pens with flushed water is an easy and clean way to handle manure Variations of this method have been adopted across much of the United States in dairy, poultry, and swine operations. Separation of solids from flushed manure by some manner is potentially important in most of these systems for several reasons:

- To remove large particles and sand that would plug or damage distribution nozzles in irrigation systems used to evenly spread the liquid over the cropping area.
- (null)

To reduce the biological loading on aerobic and anaerobic lagoons.

- To capture a fibrous product and some of the N and mineral nutrients which might be utilized in other products such as bedding for free stalls, part of the feed for cattle on maintenance diets, compost for potting material for plants, etc.

Many systems exist which will remove a portion of the solids from manure slurries. The stationary screen is most common with many new dairies experimenting with settling basins of various shapes, depths, and capacities.

Stationary screen separators take out 20 per cent to 30 per cent of the organic matter from flushed dairy manure. With very dilute flushed dairy manure, an estimate of 20 per cent removal of organic solids is probably most appropriate. Dilution also assures that almost all of the soluble nutrients will stay with the water portion. Most of the minerals and N are in soluble form.

The feeding value of this product will not support acceptable daily gains in growing ruminants. However, the manure solids could be fed as an appreciable percentage of diets for cattle which need only to maintain themselves and sustain a slow rate of gain; well-conditioned dry cows.

Screened manure solids have been used extensively for bedding in free stalls. However, management to prepare the product properly is critical.

An accepted practice seems to be to compost the solids so that internal temperatures within the pile become high enough to kill coliform bacteria.

Research has shown that even though bacteria decline to low or undetectable numbers during the composting period, bacteria often return in the bedding material in the free stalls unless there is opportunity to dry the solids in sunlight.

Even when researchers found higher bacterial counts in composted dairy waste solids bedding than on rubber mats, there was no difference in bacterial counts on teats or in the milk of cows using the two types of bedding.

They concluded that with "adequate" composting, dairy waste solids were a suitable bedding in free stalls. Many dairy farmers with excellent mastitis control programmes are using dry, screened manure solids for bedding in free stalls.

An alternative to removing solids from flushed manure with screening equipment is to design holding basins for gravity separation (settling basins). More solids can be removed with well-designed sedimentation basins than with stationary screens.

The key is the detention time of the water carrying the solids. However, the sedimented solids have much higher moisture content and are not as useful as screened solids if bedding for free stalls or composting is desired. Thus, land-spreading of these solids is the most likely method of disposal.

COMPOSTING

Composting systems have recently received much attention to facilitate exporting nutrients from dairy farms. A composting system is a modification of a conventional or solid manure handling system with the composting (treatment) process applied to the manure. Types of composting systems include windrow, bin, static pile, and aerated static pile. Major factors to be considered are the desired quality of the final product, space requirements, labour requirements, and availability of a diluent to mix with the raw waste.

Before a composting system is initiated, careful attention must be given to a market or outlet for the composted manure. Do not assume that there will be a line of people waiting to buy the product. Composting is primarily an oxidative process which removes many odorous compounds. Also, some organic solids are converted to carbon dioxide thus reducing volume, and easily volatilized nitrogen is lost. However, the final product is stable and much less odorous than the initial manure.

ESTIMATED NUTRIENT LOSSES

Even with a "tightly" managed system, there is considerable N loss through ammonia volatilization. The amount volatilized is influenced by level of N in the manure (particularly the part originating in the urine) and by the method of application. Nitrogen in urine is originally excreted in the form of urea.

Urease enzyme of bacterial origin is present almost everywhere manure is voided or stored so that N in urea is readily converted to ammonia which will be lost to the air as free ammonia unless the conditions of storage are acidic. It was estimated that 41 to 50 per cent of the manure N from lactating dairy cows is in urea or ammonia form (mostly from the urine).

This portion is potentially volatilized very rapidly. Most of the fecal N from cattle is in a more stable form; however, even organic N is freed and volatilized during anaerobic digestion. For irrigated, highly diluted manure the loss of ammonia during irrigation is often proportional to the evaporation loss of water.

Leaching losses also may occur. Application of manures outside the growing season or in amounts which exceed crop needs may result in nitrate leaching losses of 25 per cent or more of the applied N. A high utilization of N by crops can be achieved with lowered environmental risks when manures are applied at a time when crops can absorb the mineral-N and at rates that do not exceed crop needs.

Denitrification is a bacterial process which converts nitrate in solution to nitrogen gas. It is dependent upon a bacterial energy source, usually in the form of soluble organic matter, and progresses most rapidly under high moisture and/or low oxygen soil conditions. While collection and storage losses will be accounted for by sampling prior to land application, volatilization and denitrification losses after the manure leaves collection/storage are more difficult to quantify. Denitrification losses are harder to estimate on the farm but can be extensive.

POTENTIAL NUTRIENT REMOVAL BY PLANTS

One generally accepted philosophy of land application of manures is that nutrients can be applied to land in amounts slightly above the level of the nutrients removed by the crops harvested. When animal numbers are high in relation to the amount of land readily available, we need to know the maximum application rates for given soil types and crops that can be efficiently utilized by different cropping systems. We also need to use cropping systems that will take up the maximum amount of environmentally sensitive nutrients such as N and P.

A long-term research project at Tifton, Georgia was designed to identify a maximum, environmentally safe
[illegible] rate of manure nutrients when a triple-cropping
[illegible] used. Flushed dairy manure nutrients were
[illegible] centre-pivot irrigation. The cropping system
[illegible]4 bermudagrass in which corn was sod-
[illegible] spring and abruzzi rye was sod-seeded

In the Georgia experiment, large-particle manure solids were separated from the liquid with an inclined stainless steel separating screen to facilitate irrigation of the effluent. The liquid portion was applied to the cropping area at four different rates. Harvests of all crops yielded 6.2 tons or more of dry matter per acre (12,400 lbs) with N-deficient application of 214 lb N/acre with yields plateauing at 12.5 to 13.0 tons of DM/acre with manure wastewater applications of 440 lb N/ acre or more. Crop removals of N, however, continued to increase after DM yields plateaued because of luxury consumption of N, which increased CP and N concentrations of crops harvested.

Other forage crops, even legumes, like alfalfa and perennial peanut, have been proposed as being good crops for consuming large quantities of manure nutrients. When free N is available in the soil to "scavenge," legumes take up soil N in preference to fixing N from the air.

Giant elephantgrass, which has been used in field studies in Okeechobee County, Florida, gives the highest estimated P uptake. Although there may be potential for greater recovery of P in the enormous quantity of biomass harvested in giant elephantgrass than from other crops, the estimated digestible energy value of the harvested forage would be low.

The Georgia cropping system has great potential for Southern United States because: a large part of the harvest is corn silage, a high-energy forage that fits the feed needs of high producing cows; the bermudagrass forms a sod base and forage for harvest in the warm season; and rye utilizes a large amount of N during the winter season.

A cropping system tested at the University of Florida that shows promise is based on perennial peanut, a higher quality base forage than bermudagrass. Perennial peanut, although not as high yielding as bermudagrass, will utilize applied N and, additionally, may offer potential as a legume to fix some N if temporary soil deficiencies occur.

The Florida research evaluated a sod-based triple-cropping system and perennial peanut overseeded with rye in winter. These were compared with a triple-crop system of corn, forage sorghum, and rye. Note that total dry matter harvests from the corn-perennial peanut-rye system were similar to those obtained with corn-bermudagrass-rye in the Georgia experiments but somewhat less N was removed, primarily due to lesser N in the winter rye crop.

This was because of less dry matter yield and much less N content in the dry matter. Phosphorus removals on this system were 56 lb P/acre on all three N applications. The perennial peanut-rye system removed less dry matter but was an efficient scavenger of N, suggesting that some N-fixation from the legume may have taken place.

One of the major strengths of using flushed manure systems, along with irrigation, is that additional water can be applied along with fertilizer nutrients so that full response to added nutrients is possible.

Index

M

N

O

P

R

S